Independent Pr
for Parame

CW00541411

Edited by
Amanda Blaber, Hannah Morris and Andy Collen

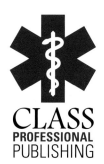

CLASS
PROFESSIONAL
PUBLISHING

This edition first published 2018

The publishers and author welcome feedback from readers of this book.

Class Professional Publishing
The Exchange, Express Park, Bristol Road, Bridgwater TA6 4RR
Email: info@class.co.uk
www.classprofessional.co.uk
Class Professional Publishing is an imprint of Class Publishing Ltd
A CIP catalogue record for this book is available from the British Library

ISBN: 9781859597873 (paperback)
ISBN: 9781859597880 (ebook)

Cover design by Hybert Design Limited, UK
Designed and typeset by Class Professional Publishing
Printed in UK by Short Run Press

Contents

About the Authors

Editors

Amanda Blaber

University of Brighton, UK

Amanda has 17 years' experience teaching in higher education institutes, with many years of emergency care experience. She contributes to the Forum for Higher Education for Paramedics and the Council of Deans Paramedic Advisory group. She is an Honorary Fellow of the College of Paramedics and is extremely proud of the literary contribution she and her colleagues have made to the education of paramedics in the UK. She has extensive knowledge and experience in curriculum design and validation processes and is a Senior Fellow of the Higher Education Academy. As a lecturer, she finds inspiration and enjoyment from teaching and endeavours to make students' learning as real and as fun as possible. She has published (alone and with colleagues) four paramedic texts, two of which are bestsellers and have resulted in further editions being written. She is committed to supporting early career writers to have the opportunity to develop their skills and experience in the publishing arena. She has been educated about 'prescribing' from her fellow editors during this process and has enjoyed learning much more about this fascinating area of practice.

Andy Collen

South East Coast Ambulance NHS Foundation Trust, UK

Andy Collen is currently a Consultant Paramedic at South East Coast Ambulance Service NHS Foundation Trust, and is also the author of *Decision Making in Paramedic Practice* (2017). Andy is the Medicines and Prescribing Project Lead for the College of Paramedics, working with NHS England and other Allied Health Professional (AHP) Professional Bodies on the proposal to extend nonmedical prescribing, including the work to introduce independent prescribing for advanced paramedics. He has been in the NHS since 1989, and progressed through a traditional ambulance service career, qualifying as a paramedic in 2000.

After qualifying as a specialist paramedic in 2006, he left the ambulance service to practice in a Walk In Centre in order to develop his skills. He returned to the ambulance service full time in 2009 to lead the specialist paramedic programmes and to work on improving professional careers and clinical leadership. He completed a MSc in 2013 and was appointed to his consultant post in 2015.

Andy sits on the Ambulance Lead Paramedic Group and the National Ambulance Urgent and Emergency Care Group. He previously contributed to the JRCALC guidelines and the UK edition of *Emergency Care in the Streets*. He undertakes sessional lectures on decision making at universities in the South East region and has presented extensively on the prescribing project across the UK. When not working in a professional capacity, Andy is a drummer and music fan. Most importantly, he enjoys spending time with his family.

Hannah Morris

University of Brighton, UK

Hannah has extensive experience as a district nurse and an advanced nurse practitioner in primary care before commencing her academic career four years ago. She is a principal lecturer and programme lead for independent prescribing in health sciences. She has 13 years' prescribing practice experience and enjoys being able to facilitate others to undertake safe and effective prescribing practice within a variety of clinical and professional roles.

Hannah has published in the field of district nursing and recognises the challenges faced by practitioners working in primary care settings and lone roles in the context of prescribing. She has worked particularly with older people and in long-term condition management in her nursing practice, and has successfully facilitated a range of practitioners to successfully complete the independent prescribing programme. She is excited to incorporate paramedics in their pivotal role as frontline practitioners into contemporary health care delivery.

Contributors

Vince Clarke

University of Hertfordshire, UK

Vince works at the University of Hertfordshire as Senior Lecturer in Paramedic Science, where he has been employed since 2016. He joined the London Ambulance Service in 1996, qualified as paramedic in 1998 and entered the Education and Development Department in 2001. He worked as part of the Higher Education team and developed in-house paramedic programmes as well as working closely with higher education partner institutions.

A Health & Care Professions Council partner since 2006, Vince has been involved in the approval of a wide range of paramedic educational programmes across the country, as well as assessing CPD submissions and sitting on Conduct and Competence Fitness to Practise panel hearings. He also works as an independent paramedic expert witness for the Court and prepares reports on breach of duty for both claimants and defendants.

Graham Harris

National Education Lead, College of Paramedics, UK

Graham has a 47-year history in pre- and out-of-hospital care which covers working in the military, the NHS, higher education and the professional body for UK paramedics. He has co-edited with Amanda Blaber the first and second editions of *Assessment Skills for Paramedics* and *Clinical Leadership for Paramedics*, and has co-authored chapters in all three editions of *Foundations for Paramedic Practice*. He has held Council, Executive and Trustee Official positions within the College of Paramedics, and for the past three years has been employed as the National Education Lead developing pre-registration and postgraduate curriculums, and other national standards for the paramedic profession

Jennifer Whibley

University of Brighton, UK

Jennifer has been a pharmacist for almost 15 years and has worked in different care settings before moving into teaching. Jennifer has been community pharmacist, worked in a range of specialities in hospital pharmacy as well as in different capacities in general practice. Throughout her career, she has had a passion for training and education and has been involved in teaching both pharmacists and a range of other healthcare professionals. She made the move to working in higher education full time in 2015, initially as a lecturer in a school of medicine and more recently as a senior lecturer of pharmacology for non-medical prescribers. She has undertaken a range of postgraduate training, including a PgDip in pharmacy practice as well as a PGCert in Teaching in Higher Education. She is also a Fellow of the Higher Education Academy. She won a place as a student to complete a placement on a national pharmacy journal and has co-authored several articles, but this is the first text she has contributed to. She has enjoyed the challenge of making a subject that some find difficult and confusing into something that learners will be able to use and apply in practice.

Acknowledgements

Very many thanks to our academic and advanced practice colleagues who provided many of the case studies and worked to a tight schedule.

Our thanks goes to Dylan Griffin, Dr Angela McAdam and Julie Ormrod.

Abbreviations and Acronyms

ADHD	attention deficit hyperactivity disorder
ADME	absorption, distribution, metabolism and elimination
ADRs	adverse drug reactions
AHPF	Allied Healthcare Professions Federation
AHPs	allied health professions
AI	artificial intelligence
AKI	acute kidney injury
ALS	advanced life support
BASICS	British Association of Immediate Care
BMJ	British Medical Journal
BNF	British National Formulary
BNFC	British National Formulary for Children
CD	controlled drug
CHM	Commission on Human Medicines
CKD	chronic kidney disease
CKS	Clinical Knowledge Summary
CMP	clinical management plan
CoP	College of Paramedics
COPD	chronic obstructive pulmonary disease
COX	Cyclooxygenase
CPD	continuing professional development
CPPD	continuing personal and professional development
CrCl	Creatinine Clearance
CRP	C-reactive protein
DHSS	Department of Health and Social Security
DMP	designated medical practitioner
DVT	deep vein thrombosis
eGFR	estimated glomerular filtration rate
eMC	Electronic Medicines Compendium
FBC	full blood count
GDPR	General Data Protection Regulation
GI	gastrointestinal

GPCRs	G-protein coupled receptors
GSL	general sales list
HAIs	hospital-acquired infections
HCPC	Health and Care Professions Council
HIV	Human Immunodeficiency Virus
HMR	Human Medicines Regulations
ICE	ideas, concerns and expectations
IP	initial profile
IT	information technology
ITU	intensive therapy unit
IV	intravenous
MECC	Making Every Contact Count
MHRA	Medicines and Healthcare products Agency
MHRA	Medicines and Healthcare products Regulatory Agency
MMR	measles, mumps, and rubella
MRSA	methicillin-resistant Staphylococcus aureus
NHS	National Health Service
NICE	National Institute of Health and Care Excellence
NPC	National Prescribing Centre
NSAID	non-steroidal anti-inflammatory drug
OTC	over-the-counter
PCD	person-centred development
PGD	Patient Group Direction
PHOF	Public Health Outcomes Framework
POMS	prescription only medicines
PSD	Patient Specific Direction
RCEM	Royal College of Emergency Medicines
RPC	Royal Pharmaceutical Council
SPC	Summary of Product Characteristics
SPS	Specialist Pharmacy Services
TB	tuberculosis
TDM	therapeutic drug monitoring
TIAs	transient ischemic attacks
U&Es	urea & electrolytes
UTI	urinary tract infection
VBG	venous blood gas
Vd	volume of distribution

Introduction

Independent prescribing for paramedics is a challenging and exciting development for the profession. As this text will present, there has been a considerable amount of hard work and diligence by key people within the College of Paramedics to get to this exciting professional threshold.

The College is clear that the independent paramedic prescribing roles only be undertaken by paramedics who are working in an advanced paramedic role; fulfil the definition of an advanced practitioner, and usually have masters level education (or who are actively working towards a Masters degree or have many years of consolidated clinical experience). Those using the term 'paramedic independent prescriber' need to have successfully completed an accredited higher education prescribing course.

In line with the above paragraph, this text has been designed to support independent paramedic prescribers, who will be new to the role and it is hoped this text will be supportive, educational and very useful.

Within the text the reader will find that many chapters contain case studies that have been provided by advanced paramedics to illustrate certain points of the individual chapters. There are 'think about' boxes in chapters which encourage the reader to consider points in more detail and apply to their own practice environment. Finally, there are 'turn to' prompts that highlight the inextricable nature of the subjects of many of the chapters.

Chapter 1
Background to Independent Prescribing for Paramedics

Andy Collen

In This Chapter

♦ Introduction
♦ Background to non-medical prescribing
♦ Overview of the prescribing mechanisms
♦ The history of independent prescribing by paramedics
♦ Prescribing roles
♦ Rationale and case of need
♦ Aims of paramedic prescribing
♦ Conclusion
♦ Key points of this chapter
♦ References

Introduction

This chapter provides an overview of non-medical prescribing in the United Kingdom (UK). It provides a historical perspective describing how prescribing has developed for non-medical healthcare practitioners in the UK and charts the journey that paramedic prescribing has taken. It includes a contemporary take on the need for paramedic prescribing in today's healthcare context and an analysis of what this can offer patients and healthcare practice.

Background to Non-medical Prescribing

Prior to changes made in the early 1990s, prescribing medicines was restricted to doctors, dentists and veterinarians. The legal basis for prescribing medicines in healthcare is described in the Medicines Act 1968 (Legislation.gov.uk, 2015), which states the legislative and practical limitations imposed on access to medicines in order to prevent harm to patients and the wider population. It provides a framework for the licensing of medicines, and clarifies the classes and schedules of medicinal products available in the UK. As with all legislation, it can be extremely challenging to navigate and provides very limited detail which can be easily interpreted by the layperson, but must be upheld to ensure legitimate and legal practice.

The basis of the law requires that the correct medicine is given to the correct patient in the right way (dose, presentation, formulation) and at the right time. As the Medicines Act regulates the administration, supply and licensing of medicines, it is important that medicines in practice be entrusted only to appropriate practitioners. It is these restrictions which in turn created an increasing number of practical issues for patients to access medicines in a timely way in a modernising healthcare system.

Non-medical prescribing was first proposed in the recommendations published in the Cumberledge Report (Department of Health and Social Security (DHSS), 1986), which suggested prescribing be undertaken by community nurses. The Crown Report written by Dr June Crown in 1989 (Crown, 1999) endorsed the recommendations made in the Cumberledge Report, and this led to the creation of specific legislation to allow nurse prescribing (Medicinal Products: Prescription by Nurses etc. Act 1992). Nurse prescribing developed over the subsequent years and paved the way for non-medical prescribing to be extended beyond nursing and pharmacists. The introduction of prescribing by allied health professions (AHPs) happened in 2013 when the physiotherapy and podiatry professions achieved independent prescribing responsibilities, following lobbying for changes to the Human Medicines Regulations (2012). This initial project led to further AHP non-medical prescribing proposals, with radiographers, dietetics and paramedics achieving independent and/or supplementary prescribing. The aims of non-medical prescribing are:

♦ to improve patients' access to treatment and advice;
♦ to make more effective use of the skills and expertise of groups of professions;
♦ to improve patient choice and convenience;
♦ to contribute to more flexible team-working across the National Health Service (NHS).

Prescribing authority by the overarching profession is described in the legislation, whereas the authority given to individual practitioners is effectively delegated to the professional regulator (which for AHPs is the Health and Care Professions Council [HCPC]). The law describes the 'appropriate practitioner' and the need to complete education commensurate to the responsibilities given to the prescriber. The role of the HCPC is therefore to approve education programmes which aspirant prescribers must undertake in order to apply to have their registration annotated. *Annotation* is the evidence of authority and is awarded to the registrant on completion of the education programme to become a prescriber, and exists only while the practitioner has a prescribing role. Where the prescriber changes their role (for example, moving into a leadership role from a clinical role), the annotation should be removed. Annotation can also be removed as part of the usual activities of the regulator, such as the result of a fitness to practice hearing.

Non-medical prescribing is now very well-established and embedded within clinical services across the country. The aims of non-medical prescribing have driven the expansion of prescribing responsibilities to other professions, including paramedics, and while these achievements are notable for the profession, the basis for prescribing is about safe and timely patient care. Paramedics have a long relationship with medicines, and the granting of independent prescribing co-exists alongside other legal mechanisms that paramedics can access (exemptions and patient group directions) and should enhance the contribution paramedics make in providing the best possible care for patients.

Overview of the Prescribing Mechanisms (Independent and Supplementary Prescribing)

Independent and supplementary prescribing is the most significant medicines mechanism that any healthcare profession can practise using, and responsibility associated with prescribing requires well-developed professional insight. One of the most challenging situations for prescribers which differs from other mechanisms is the autonomy to decide on what and when to prescribe rather than following a protocol. The constant tension between legal, ethical and practical considerations in practice applies to all medicines mechanisms open to paramedics, and highlights the trust in the profession by the establishment and patients.

Box 1.1 – Definitions of independent and supplementary prescribing

Supplementary Prescribing

The main principle of supplementary prescribing is that the patient is already known to the clinical team providing their care, and they have an existing diagnosis. A doctor will have prepared a Clinical Management Plan which lists the medicines intended for the patients care and from which a supplementary prescriber can prescribe.

Independent Prescribing

Independent prescribing is prescribing by a suitable practitioner who can provide holistic care for the patient and develop a care and treatment plan for the patient (within their area of speciality and/or competency) based on the individual aspects required to achieve that, such as physical assessment, diagnostic skills or pharmacological knowledge. Prescribing practice sometimes infers always simply adding more medicines, but in fact reality requires consideration to not prescribe and/or to de-prescribe, as well to prescribe.

Prescribing is a complex undertaking and is made more complex by the nuances of different patient groups and practice settings. Prescribing requires high levels of clinical judgement and the use of the evidence base and practice guidance to inform decisions. For paramedics, the profession has a long relationship with medicines, but its context is very much protocol-driven and based on gross symptomaticity and clinical findings to inform and direct actions. This is therefore often biased towards action, and for prescribers there is a tension between prescribing and not prescribing (and, indeed, de-prescribing), as is made clear in **Box 1.1**, where definitions are provided. Prescribing as a mechanism, while inferring a pinnacle in the hierarchy, must be seen as the most appropriate mechanism for use, and the other mechanisms should continue to be embraced (for example, using exemptions for resuscitation drugs).

The History of Independent Prescribing by Paramedics

Prescribing by paramedics as a concept originated in 2009 and progressed as far as a ministerial consultation being undertaken and published in 2010 (Department of Health, 2010a). While the consultation report was positive, the project did not progress at that time and was dormant for a number of years. The successful implementation of independent prescribing by physiotherapy and podiatry in 2013 (along with supplementary prescribing by radiographers) led to the expansion of the Allied Health Professions Medicines Programme within NHS England and included the following proposals:

♦ Use of exemptions by Orthoptists;
♦ Supplementary prescribing by Dietitians;
♦ Independent prescribing by Radiographers (expanding their supplementary prescribing status);
♦ Independent prescribing by Paramedics.

(NHS England, 2015e)

The project began in 2014 and focused initially on building a 'case of need' to describe the outline requirement and to gather sufficient support to seek ministerial approval to undertake a public consultation on the proposals. The case of need was developed and approved by the Medical and Nursing Senior Management Teams within NHS England in May 2014, and the Non-Medical Prescribing Board in the Department of Health in July of the same year. A submission to ministers was made to request the commencement of a public consultation, and this was granted in August 2014. The 12-week consultation period for the radiography and paramedic proposals took place between 26 February and 22 May 2015 (an eight-week consultation period for orthoptists and dietitians was also undertaken) and involved the publication of surveys which could be completed online. A number of engagement events were also held across the UK in the summer of 2015. The consultation for paramedics asked for a preference among five options:

♦ No change.
♦ Independent prescribing for any condition from a full formulary.
♦ Independent prescribing for specified conditions from a specified formulary.
♦ Independent prescribing for any condition from a specified formulary.
♦ Independent prescribing for specified conditions from a full formulary.

(NHS England, 2015e)

The consultation also asked for respondents to comment on the proposal to include a restricted list of controlled drugs (CDs) as part of the overall proposal (but subject to additional regulatory and legislative changes after the initial approval of independent prescribing). It also asked if paramedics should be able to mix medicines.

Across the four professions involved on the consultation, several thousand responses were received, and the vast majority were supportive of the proposals. The paramedic consultation received 536 responses, of which 96% were in favour of the proposal for independent prescribing and around 75% were in favour of Option 2 (independent prescribing for any condition from a full formulary) (NHS England 2015a, p. 23). The consultation also yielded narrative responses and included some notable support from a number of key organisations:

> We strongly support a move to independent prescribing for appropriately trained advanced paramedics. Would allow easier access to appropriate medications for patients.
>
> British Association of Immediate Care (BASICS)

> Yes. Paramedics play a vital role in the acute care pathway. Enabling advanced paramedics to independently prescribe will enable more patients to be treated in their own home and open up more roles in different care settings for the paramedics.
>
> Royal College of Emergency Medicine

> Yes. It seems eminently sensible to permit a wider group of regulated, highly qualified, trained professionals to prescribe. They are the experts in their respective fields.
>
> Public Health England
>
> (NHS England 2015a, p. 23)

Very few organisational responses provided negative responses, although two were received suggesting that supplementary prescribing would be more appropriate for paramedics, and some individual (non-organisational) responses were pointedly against.

Once concluded, approval was sought to present the proposals and the consultation findings to the Commission on Human Medicines (CHM). This was granted and the first attendance at CHM took place in October 2015. The CHM was established as a sub-committee of the Medicines and Healthcare products Regulatory Agency (MHRA) in October 2005, and was formed to advise ministers on the safety, efficacy and quality of medicinal products. Its roles were extended to also advise on the suitability of proposals for additional healthcare professions being granted prescribing responsibilities, beginning with physiotherapy and podiatry in 2012/13. Following the first meeting in October 2015, the CHM did not support the proposals for paramedic prescribing, and this decision was included in the minutes of the meeting which were published in December 2015.

The project team at NHS England, supported by the College of Paramedics (CoP) and other AHP professional bodies, sought to resolve the challenges put forward by the CHM, and permission was sought to return to the CHM to give further assurances regarding patient safety and medicines governance. In response to the importance given to safely and appropriately extended non-medical prescribing (and mindful that other proposals were being presented by radiographers and dietitians), a Technical

Working Group of the CHM was selected to hear the subsequent approach on the proposals. The meeting in 2016 was extremely positive and, while ultimately not successful, provided detail and clarity on the areas of concern, which would be worked on in the lead up to a further attendance at the CHM Technical Working Group in July 2017. At this meeting, recommendations were made to the main CHM meeting to endorse independent prescribing by paramedics:

> The Commission considered and discussed feedback from the ad hoc group on the proposals for Independent Prescribing for Paramedics ... In conclusion, the Commission endorsed the ad-hoc group's recommendations to support independent prescribing for paramedics.
>
> (CHM, 2017, p. 2)

Subsequently, a submission to ministers was made to request an amendment to the Statutory Instrument (the Human Medicines Regulations) and the legislation was laid in February 2018. On 1 April 2018, the amendment came into force legally allowing paramedics who fulfil the requirements of an 'appropriate practitioner' to undertake independent and supplementary prescribing.

While the Human Medicines Regulation 2018 amendment (Legislation.gov.uk, 2018) provides the overarching ability to become prescribers, there are other pieces of regulatory legislation which need to be amended to include paramedics:

♦ the NHS (General Medical Services Contracts) Regulations 2015 (NHS England, 2015b)
♦ the NHS (Personal Medical Services Agreement) Regulations 2015 (NHS England, 2015c)
♦ the NHS (Charges for Drugs and Appliances) Regulations 2015 (NHS England, 2015d)
♦ the NHS (Pharmaceutical and Local Pharmaceutical Services) Regulations 2013 (NHS England, 2013).

Common to all non-medical prescribing professions who need to include controlled drugs in their formulary, amendments also have to be made to the Misuse of Drugs Regulations (2001) to ensure that the additional legislative approval exists for practice involving CDs. The original proposal for paramedic independent prescribing included the ability to prescribe from a restricted list of six controlled drugs, which would be specifically cited in the amendment to the Misuse of Drugs Regulations (2001). All professions who achieve non-medical prescribing responsibilities to date have undergone a period using a restricted CD formulary. Physiotherapy and podiatry achieved independent prescribing in 2013 and began a review of their original list of CDs in 2018, and this timeframe should be anticipated for any subsequent review of paramedic CDs.

The professional bodies which lead individual professions (such as the College of Paramedics, the Chartered Society of Physiotherapy, and the Society and College of Radiographers) have a responsibility to publish practice guidance documents which provide information on the specific elements of safe practice. The professional bodies work closely to ensure that practice guidance is consistent, but each of the common aspects of practice detailed in the guidance is nuanced to the specific profession based on a range of considerations such as practice settings, underpinning competencies, patient groups and diseases treated. Practice guidance is a vitally important document which supports safe non-medical prescribing and should be read and understood as part of ongoing prescribing practice.

For any profession to achieve independent prescribing responsibilities is significant. For paramedics, this is even more significant considering the fact that professional regulation only started for paramedics 20 years ago. When compared to the other professions that have prescribing in their practice, these professions have been established for far longer and have had more opportunity to become embedded in their practice settings. Paramedics have seen an exponential increase in the opportunity to practise in ever more diverse settings and with ever-increasing trust in their abilities. This has created more and more demand for paramedics because of the care they can offer and the 'unique selling points' that the profession has. Challenges also accompany these successes, and these should not be overlooked when we consider our professional journey. Prescribing is a complex aspect of clinical practice and encompasses virtually all conceivable aspects of care planning from communication skills to diagnoses, disease knowledge, pharmacological knowledge, pharmacovigilance, care planning – the list goes on. As a profession with a long relationship with medicine as an intervention, care should be taken to look upon prescribing as a very different 'animal' – less intervention, more wrapping around the patient and their needs. Prescribing education should be taken based only on the needs of the patients you see in your role, and never as simply CPD. It is a professional way of life which exists to optimise the safe and timely access to medicines patient deserve.

Turn to **Chapter 4** for more detail regarding prescribing pharmacology.

Prescribing Roles

In order to embark on prescribing education, prescribing must be a requirement of the clinician's job role. The same is true of the process of registrant annotation with the Health and Care Professions Council; ongoing annotation is only possible where a prescribing role exists. Prescribing roles vary greatly across different professions and, in the early period of paramedic prescribing, these roles will continue to emerge. Much of the variety associated with prescribing roles originates in the practice setting; the broad scopes of practice among paramedics; patient need; and the disease seen. In many ways the notion of a prescribing role should be self-evident and clearly articulated in job descriptions, clinical service specifications, appraisals and professional development plans.

For paramedics working in clinical roles requiring independent prescribing as a core skill (such as the Advanced Clinical Practitioner model developed by the Royal College of Emergency Medicines [RCEM]) (RCEM, 2017), the development and expectation is to a large degree pre-ordained, but for other roles and practice settings, the justification for prescribing may need to emerge in order to garner support. The guidance issued by the College of Paramedics and Outline Curriculum Framework published by the Allied Healthcare Professions Federation (AHPF) (AHPF, 2017) suggest that a requirement to prescribe should form an evidential gap in practice and therefore create an issue which impacts patients' timely access to medicines. The ability to train as a prescriber from a purely legal perspective exists, but undertaking the education comes at the end of a process where the prescribing role is clarified and all of the other requirements are in place to support the transition to practice (for example, supervision, prescribing budget, audit plan, medicines governance system and pharmacist support).

Turn to **Chapter 2** for more information regarding law and ethics.

The paramedic profession has enjoyed a rapid expansion of its core role most commonly associated with ambulance services, and continues to proliferate into areas of care which may not have even been envisaged at the start of the prescribing journey in 2014. Paramedics are now working in a number of practice settings (see **Box 1.2**) and prescribing may form an important aspect of the care they provide.

Box 1.2 – Practice settings where paramedics may be employed

♦ Primary care – GP surgery
♦ Community teams (i.e. admission avoidance/long-term condition team)
♦ Emergency departments (Advanced Clinical Practitioner)
♦ Minor injury units/walk-in centres
♦ Out-of-hours services
♦ Critical care (Advanced Critical Care Practitioner)
♦ Hospice

The practice settings identified in **Box 1.2** will most commonly require full independent prescribing, but increasingly there will be opportunities for paramedics to practise using supplementary prescribing, particularly in the hospice sector and long-term condition teams in the community. Irrespective of the setting in which prescribing happens and the type of prescribing, paramedics must focus on the principles of prescribing in order to optimise medicines use and to promote the safest possible care for patients. As mentioned previously, paramedics are privileged to be able to use medicines exemptions, patient group directions, patient specific directions and, for advanced paramedics, prescribing. The range of mechanisms open to paramedics, particularly those in prescribing roles, must be respected and considered as part of the overarching approach to practice. This means that not all medicines may be prescribed, and other mechanisms may be preferred for reasons of consistency, expedience or safety. For example, when working in an ambulance trust, administering medicines during advanced life support (ALS), such as adrenaline and amiodarone, is best achieved using exemptions, with indications and dosing informed by published practice guidance (Resuscitation Council UK; European Resuscitation Council). In situations where the patient needs a medicine immediately, while prescribing in some settings may be the preference, organisational arrangements and governance may require a PGD (Patient Group Direction) or protocol to be followed. It is important to note and to reflect upon the nature of the mechanisms that paramedics can use. Compared to other legal mechanisms such as PGDs and prescribing, the use of exemptions support immediate, pro-action clinical situations such as resuscitations where the medicine choice is limited; the time to administer well defined, and the patients' need is unequivocal. Compare this to the patient for whom their medicines require optimisation as part of the provision of a new medicine. This is a significant step for paramedics who are new to the prescriber role. The approach to the episode of care and the pace of decision making is very different from more familiar scenarios in more urgent care situations.

Non-medical prescribing has inherent supervisory oversight, and this is an opportunity for paramedics to embrace and exploit a means of working across professional boundaries, in such a way that individual practice becomes consolidated and enhanced. Paramedics may have had little or no exposure to the full range of professional activities within the domains of supervision, and this may therefore feel alien initially. One of the key benefits of non-medical prescribing is the requirement to engage in supervision which is derived from other medical and non-medical prescribers. In the early years of paramedic prescribing, the individual paramedics will need to be supervised by other AHP or nurse prescribers until such time as there are sufficiently experienced paramedics in non-medical prescribing roles able to themselves become supervisors. Those undertaking prescribing education are fortunate in that they must be supervised by a doctor (designated medical practitioner [DMP]) during the course (although the requirement for the DMP to be a doctor may be reviewed in future) and so the medical model of professional guidance and oversight will be open to those paramedics. This in turn should instil a broader understanding of supervision and reflection in all areas of practice, and not just prescribing. This will benefit the paramedic, the clinical team they are working and, importantly, the patient.

 Turn to **Chapter 10** to read more about reflection and supervision.

Rationale and Case of Need

Paramedics have a long relationship with the use of medicines as part of caring for patients, starting initially with a basic range of resuscitation drugs and expanding rapidly to include intravenous fluids, analgesia, asthma medicines and glucose, with legislation broadly keeping pace with those medicines being made available as an exemption in what become established as the specific section in Schedule 17 to the Human Medicines Regulations. As the profession developed to include specialist and advanced roles, patient group directions use proliferated (possibly beyond its initial scope), resulting in a position where the capability to optimise medicines use in practice fell behind the broader capability and scope of practice of paramedics. This natural evolution was fortunate in its timing; health policy began to shift towards 'care closer to home', and this reflected the changes in health and social care designed to address the ageing population and milestones in disease management which has led to more patients living longer with more diseases (co-morbidity). The most common practice setting for paramedics, and one with the greatest synonymy, was the ambulance sector. The rapid growth in the way in which ambulance trusts approached the new challenges of the changes in demography and epidemiology coincided with very significant policy developments in the UK, which recognised that health and social care needed to evolve. For paramedics, opportunities began to emerge in other sectors as their professional profile was more widely on display. The public and other healthcare professions were aware of the role of the paramedic in resuscitation and trauma care, but had given less attention to the potential as a first contact practitioner able to make sense of complex situations and undifferentiated presentations. Paramedics undertaking postgraduate study in all areas of practice, from urgent through to critical care, were spending time on clinical placements, and this led to the start of the shift away from paramedics being associated only with ambulance services. In recent years, the proportion of paramedics working in the ambulance sector has reduced, and while the opportunities are good for paramedics, the potential loss of capability within the ambulance sector could cause problems 'downstream'.

Fortunately, health policy has been forward-thinking enough to ensure that the increasing workforce challenges which exist in many parts of healthcare are mitigated, and specific examples such as the pilot 'rotational paramedic' schemes seek to promote a retention of senior paramedic skills and experience across the ambulance and wider primary care sector.

These changes and emerging models of care and clinical practice required changes to the proposals for independent prescribing. As the project developed, it became clear that a proposal for 750 advanced paramedic prescribers in the ambulance sector needed to be expanded to reflect the wider range of practice settings in which paramedics were working and the complexity of the roles they were undertaking. Importantly, it was the lack of prescribing responsibilities that in itself began to create problems for paramedics working in advanced practice roles, which in turn drove the 'sea-change' in support for the proposals for independent prescribing by paramedics. The principles in the Five Year Forward View (NHS England, 2014), the

Francis Report 2014 and the Darzi Report 2008 all provided support to the various areas of emphasis for the expansion of non-medical prescribing (i.e. workforce, planning of services, reducing harm, promote outcomes and experience), along with the other contemporaneous publications which continues to inform health and social care policy.

There are two assumptions within the original Case of Need document developed by NHS England (2015e), which formed the basis for the ultimate development of the project supporting the proposal for paramedic prescribing. The first is the increasing trust in the paramedic profession, as evidenced by the proliferation of practice settings, which in turn was driven by increases in demand for urgent unscheduled care. The other and by far the most important consideration is patient safety. The challenges of ensuring that patients are not harmed during healthcare will always be a key focus of clinical care and health system leadership.

Aims of Paramedic Prescribing

As discussed throughout this chapter, paramedics are being regarded with increasing trust and confidence in their practice in response to changing patient need. They have demonstrated the ability to provide excellent care in the first contact role for patients presenting with urgent, undifferentiated needs through to patients needing critical care, and responding to the context of this range of acuity whether the patient encounter is short (such as in ambulance settings) or more continuous (such as in primary care) and how this impacts on the various facets of prescribing. Paramedics continue to demonstrate their unique 'selling point' and have maintained their identity and the nuances of the profession's increasingly multi-professional workforce, to the benefit of patients. Some of the questions raised during the project to realise prescribing by paramedics included: 'Why do we need more non-medical prescribers?'. It is the articulation of the aims of paramedic prescribing that allows this question to be answered. All clinicians are able to meet the needs of patients in their areas of speciality. While there has been some broad specialisation in paramedic practice, one questions whether paramedics remain one of the last few remaining generalists, perhaps an extended or advanced/expert generalist (Benner, 1984), but, nonetheless, a generalist in its truest sense. Patients with complex diseases need specialist medical and nursing and therapies care. Where patients experience a sudden or unexpected health problem (or even an anticipated problem), they often turn to paramedics who respond to them following a 999 call, see them in the GP practice or out-of-hours centre, walk-in centre or the emergency departments. Therefore, the aim of paramedic prescribing is to 'fill the need' that was being experienced and to 'close the gap' between the rest of the paramedic skill-set and the ability to provide focused pharmacological intervention. **Case Study 1.1** highlights the resources and time wasted when prescribing is not an option.

Case Study 1.1

You are working as part of a community respiratory team and have been on duty since 06:00 on Saturday morning. At 09:15 you receive call from your ambulance colleagues who have responded to a 68-year-old male with shortness of breath and who felt that this patient required antibiotic treatment. They received their initial call at 07:45 and you agree to see the patient after completing your current visit, arriving at 10:45.

HPC: 2/7 history of increasing shortness of breath on exertion with a productive cough. No chest pain

PMH: recent diagnosis of COPD, waiting specialist review next week for management plan

Allergies: penicillin

DH: Salbutamol (with spacer)

SH: lives with wife

SE: denies chest pain, no fever, no chills, no confusion, no pursed lips, no central or peripheral oedema or cyanosis, no use of accessory muscles, activities of daily living slightly reduced.

OE: HR 112 beats per minute (bpm)

BP 135/85 mmHg

Blood glucose 5.7 mmols

RR 26 breaths per minute (bpm)

Temp 38.3 °C

SpO_2 95%

IMP: infective exacerbation of COPD chest infection

Plan: antibiotics, oral corticosteroids, discharge to care of wife, review by specialist 3/7.

As a paramedic working with the community team, your current scope of practice allows you to supply specific medicines via a PGD. You currently have the choice of two antibiotic PGDs that are indicated for chest infections. Firstly, amoxicillin, which is contra-indicated due to the patient's previous history of severe allergic reactions and, secondly, clarithromycin, which is also contra-indicated. Following National Institute of Health and Care Excellence (NICE) guidelines, this patient should receive doxycycline. All the other members of your team are prescribers, giving them the authority to prescribe the most appropriate medication to the patient in a timely manner. Your only option is to call another member of your team to come along and carry out an assessment and prescribe the medication.

Your colleague arrives three hours later and prescribes doxycycline and a course of oral steroids. In total, this patient saw both a responder and an ambulance crew (paramedic and technician) along with two registered HCPs from therespiratory team. The time taken from the point of the first consultation to the patient receiving the medication that he needed was over seven hours.

Prescribing in the context of paramedic practice should be seen as filling a gap in capability rather than 'bolting on' an additional element to practice, whilst being mindful that much of the support for the proposal to introduce prescribing for advanced paramedics began to be seen as an imperative rather than solely a professional ambition. Paramedic prescribing aims to be complementary rather than disruptive, duplicative or to displace other professions. Where the patient's needs exceed the skills and core scope of practice of a paramedic, referral back to their specialist care team will still happen. It is also worth noting the scale of independent prescribing by paramedics. The initial case of need described 750 paramedics being trained within 5 years (NHS England, 2015e), from a professional register of around 25,000. When you compare this to the nursing profession who have around 690,000 registrants and over 55,000 with a prescribing qualification, there are more than twice as many nurse prescribers as there are paramedics in the UK.

The aims of paramedic prescribing are common to all non-medical and medical prescribers: to provide patients with safe and timely access to the medicines they need. This aim extends to working in partnership with patients, their families and carers, and other health and social care professionals.

Conclusion

The journey to achieving prescribing responsibilities for paramedics began in 2009, and while the law changed in 2018, it will take many more years to fully realise the potential of prescribing by paramedics, and further evaluation will be needed to evidence the benefits becoming fully embed across all practice settings. Conceptually, non-medical prescribing is completely embedded in healthcare practice. While the multi-professional approach to prescribing education/training is central to the ethos of non-medical prescribing, there is by its very nature a requirement to ensure that the individual professions' identity is nuanced to the scope of practice and models of care for those professions.

Paramedic prescribing represents a further legal mechanism available to paramedics, along with exemptions and the use of PGDs, as well as the administration of medicines previously prescribed and dispensed.

Case Study 1.2

A 40-year-old female (Mrs B) self-presents to the Emergency Department (ED) complaining of a sudden onset of right upper quadrant pain (RUQ), with nausea, vomiting and a fever. The triage nurse notices the patient's unwell appearance and distressed demeanour, and brings her immediately into the nursing assessment room, where the Advanced Clinical Practitioner (Advanced Paramedic) is asked to urgently review the patient.

During the initial consultation, Mrs B reports an abrupt onset of RUQ pain approximately one hour after consuming a meal the previous night and, although in significant discomfort, managed to retire to bed having taken some simple over-the-counter analgesia, namely paracetamol and ibuprofen. However, the pain intensified and had awoken her from sleep during the early hours of the morning.

Using the mnemonic SOCRATES, her pain was assessed. Mrs B described the onset of pain as initially sharp in nature scoring 7/10, which had progressively become more constant with spasmodic intensities and radiated through to her back – now 9/10. She had now developed significant nausea, vomiting and low-grade fever. On further questioning, Mrs B confirms that she had suffered a similar episode a year or so ago which she attended hospital for and, following an ultrasound scan which confirmed the presence of multiple small calculi in her gall bladder, a diagnosis of biliary colic was made. Her pain during this prior admission was managed with opiate analgesia and the non-obstructing stone was subsequently passed without surgical intervention, and she was discharged home following an overnight stay in hospital. She confirms that she has no other significant past medical or surgical history, takes no regularly prescribed or over-the-counter medicines, and has no known drug or environmental allergies. She is a non-smoker, infrequently consumes alcohol, denies recreational drug use and is a housewife.

The immediate presentation was suggestive of cholecystitis secondary to biliary colic, and the presence of a now-obstructing gallstone was highly likely. The evidence-based treatment for a patient suffering with this condition would typically include the administration of intravenous medications, including: analgesia (commonly opiates), an anti-emetic, a smooth muscle relaxant, intravenous fluid therapy and the consideration of antibiotic administration to treat infections within the gall bladder and prevent abdominal sepsis. The intravenous route for these medicines was preferred due to the persistent nausea and vomiting experienced by the patient during her initial consultation. This treatment regime is evidenced by local Trust guidance and by the National Institute of Health and Care Excellence (NICE, 2017) guidelines on the management of acute cholecystitis.

Any delay in accessing such medicines may cause Mrs B to experience worsening pain or nausea, prolonged distress and increased risk of developing sepsis. In some Trusts, a small number of these medicines are available through other mechanisms, such as Patient Group Directions (PGDs). However, medicine supply and administration under this mechanism is often restrictive by nature and mandates that the clinician using the PGD must prepare and administer all the medicines personally, rather than being able to prescribe and delegate the administration to nursing colleagues, ensuring that parallel tasks are being undertaken without delay to optimise timely patient care delivery. Crown (1999) suggested that there is a 'growing expectation from patients that they will experience a seamless service with the minimum number of contacts with different health professionals consistent with patient safety' – a notion which appears increasingly prevalent almost two decades later within a modern healthcare setting. There is also a distinct lack of consistency in medicine provision within many multi-disciplinary teams, and when used in isolation or interchangeably, these mechanisms are often inherently flawed; one example of this would be the restrictive nature of PGDs, many of which may adversely affect patient care, hamper departmental efficiency and initiate a process of third-party prescribing of medicines.

This patient's presentation is undoubtedly within the scope of practice of an Advanced Clinical Practitioner (Advanced Paramedic). However, in the absence of a suitable PGD or prescriber, the responsible clinician may need to enlist the help of a fellow colleague to prescribe the required medicines who may never have seen or examined the patient they intend to prescribe for. Third-party prescribing is commonly undertaken by a doctor, dentist or other non-medical prescriber in the supply of medicines in a variety of clinical settings, despite this falling short of 'best practice'. In such cases the prescribing clinician must always satisfy themselves that the prescribing decisions are correct and that the medicines of choice are appropriate, with clear lines of professional accountability and responsibility; this can be difficult as it is wholly reliant upon a fellow colleague's accurate clinical diagnosis and proposed management plan. Third-party prescribing is not advocated by professional bodies such as the Nursing and Midwifery Council, the General Medical Council or the Health and Care Professions Council. Advanced Clinical Practitioners (Advanced Paramedics) in possession of prescribing rights would be able to facilitate safe and effective holistic care without the involvement of a third-party prescriber to complete a care episode, thereby enhancing departmental efficiencies and patient/prescriber safety, and engendering greater professional autonomy in many clinical settings.

Key Points of This Chapter

- ♦ A summary of the background to non-medical prescribing in the UK and how the practice and the law have evolved to allow paramedic prescribing in contemporary healthcare has been provided.
- ♦ The roles that paramedic prescribers will be undertaking in practice and what this can contribute to improving the experience and outcomes for patients in contemporary healthcare have been highlighted.
- ♦ Work is still needed to ensure that paramedic prescribing reflects the needs of practice contexts.

References and Further Reading

Allied Health Professional Federation (AHPF) (2017). *Outline Curriculum Framework for Education Programmes (Prescribing)*. Available at: http://www.ahpf.org.uk/files/Online%20Curriculum%20Framework.pdf [last accessed 4 July 2018].

Benner, P. (1984). *From Novice to Expert*. Menlo Park, CA: Addison-Wesley.

Commission on Human Medicines (CHM) (2017). *Commission on Human Medicines (CHM) and Expert Advisory Group (EAG) Final Summary Minutes*. Available at: https://app.box.com/s/jv487awvqzzsrdql0o34h9gg350ceyd4 [last accessed 4 July 2018].

Crown, J. (1999). *Review of Prescribing, Supply & Administration of Medicines. A report on the supply and administration of medicines under Group Protocols*. London: Department of Health.

Darzi, A. (2008). *High Quality Care for All NHS Next Stage Review Final Report*. London: The Stationery Office. Available at: https://www.gov.uk/government/uploads/system/uploads/attachment_data/file/228836/7432.pdf [last accessed 26 June 2018].

Department of Health (2010a). *Proposals to Introduce Prescribing Responsibilities for Paramedics*. Available at: http://webarchive.nationalarchives.gov.uk/20121013032656/http://www.dh.gov.uk/prod_consum_dh/groups/dh_digitalassets/@dh/@en/documents/digitalasset/dh_114384.pdf [last accessed 4 July 2018].

Department of Health (2010b). *The Chief Health Professions Officer's Ten Key Roles for Allied Health Professionals*. Available at: http://www.acprc.org.uk/Data/Resource_Downloads/10_key_roles.pdf [last accessed 4 July 2018].

Department of Health (2012). *Human Medicines Regulations (2012)*. Available at: http://www.legislation.gov.uk/uksi/2012/1916/contents/made [last accessed 4 July 2018].

Department of Health and Social Security (DHSS) (1986). *Neighbourhood Nursing: A focus for care. Report of the community nursing review Cumberledge Report*. London: HMSO.

Fawdon, H. and Adams, J. (2013). Advanced clinical practitioner role in the emergency department. *Nursing Standard*, 28(16): 48–51.

Francis, R. (2013). .*Report of the Mid Staffordshire NHS Foundation Trust Public Inquiry*. London: The Stationery Office.

Gov.uk (2014). *Helping People to Find and Stay in Work*. Available at: https://www.gov.uk/government/policies/helping-people-to-find-and-stay-in-work [last accessed 4 July 2018].

Health and Care Professions Council (2013). *Standards for Prescribers*. Available at: http://www.hcpc-uk.org/assets/documents/10004160Standardsforprescribing.pdf [last accessed 1 January 2018].

The King's Fund (2014). *Long-Term Conditions and Multi-morbidity*. Available at: http://www.kingsfund.org.uk/time-to-think-differently/trends/disease-and-disability/long-term-conditions-multi-morbidity [last accessed 4 July 2018].

Legislation.gov.uk (1992). *Medicinal Products: Prescription by Nurses etc. Act 1992*. Available at: https://www.legislation.gov.uk/ukpga/1992/28/contents [last accessed 10 July 2018].

Legislation.gov.uk (2001). *The Misuse of Drugs Regulations 2001*. Available at: http://www.legislation.gov.uk/uksi/2001/3998/contents/made [last accessed 4 July 2018].

Legislation.gov.uk (2012). *The Human Medicines Regulations 2012*. Available at: http://www.legislation.gov.uk/uksi/2012/1916/regulation/8/made [last accessed 4 July 2018].

Legislation.gov.uk (2015). *Medicines Act 1968*. Available at: http://www.legislation.gov.uk/ukpga/1968/67/contents [last accessed 4 July 2018].

Legislation.gov.uk (2018). *The Human Medicines (Amendment) Regulations 2018*. Available at: http://www.legislation.gov.uk/uksi/2018/199/pdfs/uksi_20180199_en.pdf [last accessed 4 July 2018].

Murray, K. (2013). Paramedic practitioners are key to easing the crisis in A&E. *The Guardian*, 13 November. Available at: http://www.theguardian.com/society/2013/nov/13/a-e-crisis-paramedic-practitioners-patients-home [last accessed 4 July 2018].

National Institute of Health and Care Excellence (NICE) (2017). 'Cholecystitis – acute'. Revised January 2017. Available at: https://cks.nice.org.uk/cholecystitis-acute#!scenario.

NHS England (2013a). *NHS (Pharmaceutical and Local Pharmaceutical Services) Regulations 2013*. Available at: https://www.legislation.gov.uk/uksi/2013/349/introduction/made [last accessed 23 January 2018].

NHS England (2013b). *Transforming Urgent and Emergency Care Services in England*. London: NHS England.

NHS England (2014). *Five Year Forward View*. Available: https://www.england.nhs.uk/five-year-forward-view/ [last accessed August 2018].

NHS England (2015a). *Summary of the Responses to the Public Consultation on Proposals to Introduce Independent Prescribing by Paramedics across the United Kingdom*. Available at: https://www.england.nhs.uk/wp-content/uploads/2016/02/Paramedics-summary-consult-responses.pdf [last accessed 4 July 2018].

NHS England (2015b). *The National Health Service (General Medical Services Contracts) Regulations 2015*. Available at: https://www.legislation.gov.uk/uksi/2015/1862/contents/made [last accessed 4 July 2018].

NHS England (2015c). *NHS (Personal Medical Services Agreement) Regulations 2015.* Available at: https://www.legislation.gov.uk/uksi/2015/1879/contents/made [last accessed 4 July 2018].

NHS England (2015d). *NHS (Charges for Drugs and Appliances) Regulations 2015.* Available: https://www.legislation.gov.uk/uksi/2015/570/contents/made [last accessed 4 July 2018].

NHS England (2015e). *Consultation on Proposals to Introduce Independent Prescribing by Paramedics across the United Kingdom.* Available at: https://www.engage.england. nhs.uk/consultation/independent-prescribing-paramedics/user_uploads/consult-indpndnt-prescrbng-paramedics.pdf [last accessed 6 June 2018].

Parliament (2010). *The Ageing Population.* Available at: http://www.parliament.uk/ business/publications/research/key-issues-for-the-new-parliament/value-for-money-in-public-services/the-ageing-population [last accessed 6 June 2018].

Royal College of Emergency Medicine (RCEM) (2017). *Advanced Clinical Practitioner Curriculum and Assessment.* Available at: https://www.rcem.ac.uk//docs/Training/ EM%20ACP%20curriculum%20V2%20Final.pdf [last accessed 6 June 2018].

Royal Pharmaceutical Society (2016). *A Competency Framework for All Prescribers.* Available at: https://www.rpharms.com/Portals/0/RPS%20document%20library/Open%20 access/Professional%20standards/Prescribing%20competency%20framework/ prescribing-competency-framework.pdf [last accessed 26 January 2018].

Swann, G., Chessum, P., Fisher J., Cooke M. (2013). An autonomous role in emergency departments. *Emergency Nurse,* 21(3): 13–15.

Chapter 2
Law and Ethics

Hannah Morris

In This Chapter

- ◆ Introduction
- ◆ Prescribing
- ◆ Scope of prescribing practice
- ◆ Indemnity insurance
- ◆ Legislation and prescribing
- ◆ Licensing of medicines
- ◆ Legal considerations
- ◆ Ethical considerations
- ◆ Good practice considerations
- ◆ Controlled drugs
- ◆ Evidence-based practice
- ◆ Conclusion
- ◆ Key points of the chapter
- ◆ References

Introduction

This chapter will outline the legislation and legal aspects that support paramedic prescribers in practice. Key legal and ethical concepts related to prescribing practice will be explored. Utilising evidence-based practice for safe and effective prescribing practice will be discussed.

Prescribing

Prescribing is defined as the advice and authorisation to use a medicine from the British National Formulary (BNF) and often includes the writing and issuing of a prescription (HCPC, 2018).

There are differing legal systems that govern prescribing throughout each country in the UK and paramedic prescribers should be familiar with local legal systems.

In English law there are two types of prescribers who can prescribe medicines from the BNF. These are independent prescribers and supplementary prescribers; see **Boxes 2.1** and **2.2** for definitions.

Box 2.1 – Definition of independent prescribers

Independent prescribers are those who are accountable and responsible for the assessment and treatment of new or previously diagnosed conditions and the decisions made as part of a clinical treatment plan, which may include prescribing (BNF, 2017). Independent prescribers can prescribe, stop or adjust any medicine from the BNF for patients in their care within their scope of practice.

Box 2.2 – Definition of supplementary prescribers

Supplementary prescribers work in partnership with a medical prescriber (such as a doctor or a dentist) and can implement the commencement, titration or de-prescribing of certain medicines for pre-determined patients within a clinical management plan, with the patients' consent (BNF, 2017). This means that supplementary prescribers can prescribe a range of identified medicines for certain patients within their scope of practice, with the support of a medical prescriber who writes a clinical management plan for the supplementary prescriber to follow.

In England from 1 April 2018, legislation was changed to allow some registered paramedics, working at an advanced practice level, to become independent and supplementary prescribers following a post-registration education programme that is approved by the HCPC, in conjunction with the HCPC 'standards of prescribing practice' (HCPC, 2016). Once the education programme is completed, the paramedic can annotate their prescribing qualification against their registration in order to practise as a prescriber.

Education programmes approved by the HCPC include training and preparation in competencies to undertake independent and supplementary prescribing. Therefore, if you are annotated as an independent paramedic prescriber on the HCPC register, you will also be annotated as a supplementary prescriber (College of Paramedics, 2018a). This may be of use when you are developing your scope of prescribing practice into new disease areas or in prescribing a new range of drugs. Using a clinical management plan as a supplementary prescriber could also be of use to you should you move into a new role or speciality and take your prescribing qualification with you. This will help you develop a new scope of prescribing practice in a new field of practice in a supportive context.

Scope of Prescribing Practice

Independent and supplementary prescribing for paramedics has been introduced to support and enhance the delivery of care to patients in a range of healthcare settings, and will be undertaken by paramedics in advanced roles. Just because the paramedic is working in an advanced practice role it does not mean they are 'entitled to be' or 'should be' independent prescribers. The role being undertaken by the advanced paramedic requires assessment to deem whether prescribing is an essential part of the role and therefore should be part of the job description. Where prescribing is identified as an essential aspect of the clinical role, advanced paramedics will be required to undertake an accredited independent prescribing course at a higher education institution (College of Paramedics, 2018a).

Advanced Practice

Before working at an 'advanced practice' level the paramedic should be mindful of the varying uses of the title. NHS Wales (2018:7) make a valid point about the development of advanced roles 'The range of titles and the varied meanings attributed to those titles, has led to a lack of clarity regarding what an 'Advanced Practitioner' actually is'.

Each of the UK nations has defined an **advanced practitioner**. NHS Scotland (2016: 1) defines an advanced practitioner as: 'an experienced and highly educated healthcare professional who manages the complete care for the person in their care, not solely any specific condition. Advanced practice is a level of practice, rather than a type or speciality of practice'. Whilst Health Education England (2016) defines practitioners working at an advanced level as:

> Healthcare professionals educated to master's level in Advanced Clinical Practice and have developed the skills and knowledge to allow them to take on expanded roles and scope of practice caring for patients.

What is perhaps more useful, is to explore the characteristics, role boundaries and requirements which each of the three NHS agree are essential to the practitioner working at an advanced level of practice;

♦ Advanced practice should be viewed as a 'level of practice' rather than a specific role.
♦ Advanced practice has four pillars of practice as part of the core role and function: clinical practice, leadership, facilitation of learning and evidence research and development.
♦ Masters level 7 education must underpin all Advanced Practitioner role development
♦ All Advanced Practitioners should have developed their skills and theoretical knowledge to the same standards, and should be empowered to make high level and complex decisions.
♦ Advanced Practitioner roles are applicable across all areas of practice and include staff working in clinical, education, management and leadership roles.
♦ Organisations and individual Advanced Practitioners must ensure appropriate evaluation of roles.

- Workforce planning processes across NHS organisations will identify how and where advanced practice roles are required.
- Advanced Practitioners represent a senior resource within the workforce and robust governance must be embedded to ensure patient safety.

As is highlighted in this list, advanced practice includes complex decision making and high levels of autonomy, this allow for the analysis and synthesis of complex problems across settings for the enhancement of patient experience and improved outcomes.

 Turn to **Chapter 5** for more theory on decision-making information.

As a paramedic prescriber, the College of Paramedics (2018a) identifies that you must have the sufficient education and training and competence to undertake the following in order to undertake safe and effective prescribing practice:

- Assess a patient's clinical condition.
- Undertake a through history, including medical history and medication history.
- Diagnose when necessary.
- Decide on management of the presenting condition and whether to prescribe or not and/or to refer on.
- Identify the appropriate products of medication as required.
- Advise the patient on the risks, benefits and outcomes of any intervention or prescription.
- Prescribe if the patient agrees.
- Monitor the patient's condition, including any response to any medicine prescribed.
- Give lifestyle advice where appropriate.
- Refer on where appropriate.

The College of Paramedics (2018a) provides a definition of the scope of independent prescribing for paramedic practice; see **Box 2.3**.

Box 2.3 – Definition of the scope of independent prescribing for paramedic practice

The paramedic independent prescriber may prescribe any licensed medicine from the BNF, within national and local guidelines for any condition within the practitioner's area of expertise and competence in diagnosing and treating patients with urgent health needs.

(College of Paramedics, 2018, p. 8)

Your scope of prescribing practice will relate to the areas in which you are safe and competent to prescribe. Your personal scope of prescribing practice should be identified with your employer and non-medical prescribing lead. The paramedic prescriber should identify which groups of patients you will be prescribing for, such as neonates, children, adults or older people. You will also need to identify which conditions you will be treating within your scope of prescribing practice. This can be quite generic (for example, in the area of general practice) or quite specific if you are working in a particular speciality such as cardiology. Your scope in general practice may include diabetes, asthma, low-grade infection management and skin conditions. You would then need to identify the group of medicines you intend to use within your scope of prescribing practice: for example, antidiabetic medication, inhalers and steroids, antibiotics, emollients, steroid creams and ointments.

An example of a scope of prescribing document is provided in **Figure 2.1**; however, each organisation will have its own. It is important to include one of these in your supervision or appraisal processes as a new paramedic prescriber. You can review your scope of prescribing practice as your confidence and competence in prescribing develops. You are not limited to the disease areas of medicines you identify at the start of your prescribing practice, and this will develop as your scope of prescribing practice does. You should only ever prescribe medicines that you have an in-depth understanding of, and are competent to prescribe and that are within your scope of prescribing practice. You should not feel obliged to prescribe anything you do not have a comprehensive knowledge of, even if this has been prescribed for your patient previously, especially if it is outside of your scope of prescribing practice, as you will be accountable for this action.

Key point!

You must only prescribe in the areas in which you are knowledgeable and skilled to do so safely.

You must also only prescribe in the areas in which your employer has agreed that you can do so, where this is safe to do so and you have the required employee and prescribing insurances in place.

As a paramedic prescriber, your role is to continue to facilitate multi-professional working in the care of patients. This should be done within your professional role and core competency, and prescribing for patients should not be done to make up for a 'shortfall' in other prescribers in practice settings (College of Paramedics, 2018a).

Your prescribing practice and trends can also be reviewed using a scope of prescribing practice document, similar to the example shown in **Figure 2.1**. Of course, you can and should review and reflect on your own practice, but it will be reviewed during your appraisal process and prescribing practice review, when exploring your ePACT prescribing data.

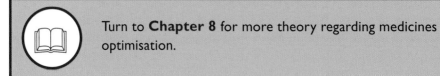

Turn to **Chapter 8** for more theory regarding medicines optimisation.

Figure 2.1 – Example of the scope of a prescribing practice document

Scope of prescribing practice		
Prescriber's name		
Job title		
Disease area(s) you will be prescribing for (Please list)		
Age group(s) you will be prescribing for (Tick as appropriate)	Neonates	
	Children and young people	
	Adults	
	Elderly	
Groups of medicines you will be prescribing (please list)		

Prescriber's signature ....

Date ....

Manager/Non-Medical Prescribing (NMP) lead signature........................

Date ....

The College of Paramedics (2018a) remains clear that as a prescriber, your scope of prescribing practice must fall within the scope of paramedic practice and be based on your practice setting. As a paramedic prescriber, you will not be permitted to prescribe outside of the UK. As a paramedic prescriber, you are also not permitted to prescribe for animals.

Indemnity Insurance

Since 2014, the HCPC has required registrants to have proof of indemnity insurance. Indemnity insurance as a prescriber may be provided within your employment contract, or you may have to source this separately. For your safety and that of your patients, it is essential that you are clear on this for your role before you commence prescribing. Paramedics practising privately or in the independent sector must ensure that their indemnity insurance is adequate for the role and practice being undertaken. Regardless of the source of the insurance, to undertake prescribing practice, and for the insurance to be valid, the paramedic must hold a valid prescribing qualification and be annotated as a prescriber on the HCPC register. Therefore, you are not permitted to prescribe until your prescribing qualification has been annotated and is visible on the HCPC register.

It is also essential to ensure that your prescribing role is evident within your job description and job role specification. This will ensure employer liability as well as that the indemnity insurance is valid.

Legislation and Prescribing

Independent prescribing for paramedics has been preceded by nurses and other allied health professionals. Since 1992, community nurses have been able to prescribe from a very limited formulary once they have completed the education and training process (Department of Health, 1989). Legislation evolved to allow some of these nurses to undertake training to prescribe from an extended formulary in 2003–2005. In 2006, the law was changed to allow nurses to undertake independent prescribing. For these historical reasons, much of the literature that allied health professionals are using now, such as practice portfolios of evidence, have been adapted from advanced nursing documents. The same applies to definitions and core requirements for advanced practice roles. In due course, Pharmacists and allied health professionals followed suit and are able to independently prescribe when working in advanced roles that require them to do so. In 2018, following a rigorous process led by the College of Paramedics, paramedics also became able to undertake the education and training to independently prescribe (College of Paramedics 2018a).

The Human Medicines Regulations (2012) provides an update to the Medicines Act (1968). These law statutes ensure that the evaluation and manufacture of medicines, and the sale and supply of medicines are regulated to keep people as safe as possible. The Human Medicines Regulations (HMR) also classify medicines for supply. These are detailed in **Table 2.1**.

Table 2.1 – The Human Medicines Regulations classification of medicines for supply

General Sales List (GSL) Medicines
A GSL medicine is deemed by the licensing authority to be on general sale. These medicines do not require a prescription or supervision from a pharmacist to be sold and are readily available in retail outlets. For example, paracetamol, ibruprofen.
Pharmacy (P) Medicines
This category of medicines can be sold without a prescription, but only under the supervision of a pharmacist. For example, hydrocortisone 1%, co-codamol.
Prescription Only Medicines (POMs)
These medicines are only available on prescription from a recognised and professionally annotated prescriber. For example Amoxicillin, Fluoxetine.
Patient Group Directions (PGDs)
A PGD is not a classification of a medicine, but an exemption of how medicines can be supplied. This is a written direction that relates to the 'sale, supply and administration of a description or class of medicinal product' (HMR 2012). A PGD enables named, authorised and registered health professionals to administer medicines to pre-defined groups of patients without a prescription so that patents have safe and speedy access to the medicines they need. A PGD should be drawn up by a multi-professional group, including a medical prescriber (doctor or dentist) and a pharmacist with representation from the professional group who will be administering medicines under the PGD, such as a nurse or paramedic (Health Education England 2016).
Patient Specific Directions (PSD)
A PSD is a written instruction by a registered and annotated prescribing professional for medicines to be supplied and/or administered to a named patient. It can be completed by an independent paramedic prescriber and may include drug authorisation charts (England 2016).

Licensing of Medicines

The Medicines and Healthcare Products Regulatory Agency (MHRA) is an executive agency that regulates the medicines, medical devices and blood components for transfusion in the UK. It provides a valid marketing authorisation for the use of medicines in the UK. This valid marketing authorisation was formally known as a Product Licence. This gives a medicine a licence for use in its indicated treatments. Paramedic prescribers will be able to prescribe any licensed medicine for any medical condition within their competence and scope of practice.

Unlicensed Use

Unlicensed drugs refer to medicines that does not hold a MHRA valid marketing authorisation, but are listed in the BNF. In general, the BNF will only list medicines that are supported by a valid marketing authorisation. Where there is an unlicensed medicine in the BNF, this is indicated in square brackets after the entry (BNF, 2017). Paramedic prescribers are NOT permitted to independently prescribe unlicensed medicines. However, if as a paramedic prescriber you prescribe as a supplementary prescriber and an unlicensed medicine is included in a clinical management plan, then you can prescribe the unlicensed medicine in this context.

If you do prescribe an unlicensed medicine within a clinical management plan, the College of Paramedics' guidance on prescribing practice (2018) stipulates that you will need to ensure:

♦ you are satisfied that an alternative licensed product would not meet the patient's needs
♦ you are satisfied that there is a sufficient evidence base for using the unlicensed medicine to demonstrate safety and efficacy
♦ that you record the medicine prescribed and the reason for using an unlicensed product in the patient notes
♦ you can clearly explain to the patient if and why you will be prescribing an unlicensed medicine.

Off label

The term 'off label' refers to the use of a medicine that has a valid marketing authorisation, but is administered via a route (for example, sublingual, orally, rectally) or way that is outside of the licensed indication of the product. This may also be referred to as 'off licence'.

Paramedic prescribers may prescribe medicines off label/off licence. This is for use outside of their licensed indications. However, they must accept clinical, professional and legal responsibility for doing so. Paramedic prescribers must only prescribe off label when it is accepted clinical practice and for any medical condition within their clinical competence and scope of prescribing practice. You must only prescribe off label with the patient's informed consent.

The College of Paramedics (2018a) recommends that when prescribing off label, you should:

♦ be satisfied that a licensed alternative is not available, which includes your proposed usage within its summary of product characteristics
♦ be satisfied there is a sufficient evidence base for using the medicine in the off label way
♦ record the medicine prescribed and the reasons for prescribing off label in the patient's notes
♦ explain to the patient why you are prescribing this medicine off label.

An example of prescribing off label: metformin is licensed for use in diabetes. It is also accepted clinical practice to use metformin in the treatment for polycystic ovary syndrome; however, the marketing authorisation does not include polycystic ovary syndrome in its indications of use. Therefore, prescribing metformin for polycystic ovary syndrome would be off label.

It is often necessary to prescribe off label in paediatric practice as medicines are often not licensed for use in children. This is due to the lack of clinical trials undertaken in children due to ethical reasons. You must explain any off label prescribing to parents or guardians and apply the same principles for prescribing in adults. You must also refer to the BNF for children and other appropriate guidelines before making any decisions in prescribing for children.

Legal Considerations

There are legal and ethical considerations to paramedic independent prescribing.

Accountability

As a professional and as an independent prescriber, you are accountable for your own prescribing decisions; this includes all actions and omissions. This accountability cannot be delegated and you will be fully responsible for all of the prescribing process. You must only prescribe within your own scope of practice, competence and experience, and in line with the HCPC standards for proficiency, ethics and prescribing. As a paramedic prescriber, you must demonstrate competence and evidence to support your ongoing prescribing practice in line with the College of Paramedics Career Framework (3rd ed. (2015)).

As a paramedic prescriber, you must only prescribe for patients who you have assessed and for who you have made the prescribing decision. You should inform patients that you are an independent non-medical paramedic prescriber and that you can only prescribe within your scope of prescribing practice and that there may be some circumstances when you need to refer on to another professional. In primary care, you should only prescribe using an FP10 prescription pad which has your own individual HCPC number on it. Accountability for the prescription is with the prescriber who has prescribed the medicines (College of Paramedics, 2018a).

Most NHS organisations now use local formularies in practice. This is to ensure evidence-based and cost effiency in prescribing practice. Some NHS organisations will only allow you to prescribe within this formulary, despite your independent prescribing status; some will allow you to prescribe outside of the formulary if you are able to demonstrate a clear rationale for doing so. Any restrictions placed upon you through a formulary would only apply while you are working with that employer.

If you move practice area, or move to work with a new employer, you may need to undertake further training and education if you wish to prescribe in a new speciality. Your new employer may wish to assess your competency as a prescriber before they support your prescribing in practice. If you undertake prescribing practice outside of employment, for example as an independent practitioner in the aesthetics industry, you will need to ensure you have completed the full training required and hold your own indemnity insurance. You will need to ensure you have the skills, knowledge and competence to prescribe in this area before doing so. If your practice pr prescribing practice is called in to question outside of your regular paramedic prescribing role, this will have implications for all your practice roles.

If there are any restrictions placed on your practice by the HCPC, it is your responsibility to inform your employer and/or insurance providers of any implications this may have on your ability to prescribe in practice (College of Paramedics, 2018a).

Consent

You must explain your role as an independent paramedic prescriber to the patient. You will need to explain that you are able to prescribe within your own scope of prescribing practice and that there may be circumstances where you will need to refer them on to another healthcare professional. You should provide the patient with all the information regarding your prescribing decision so that they are able to provide informed consent to any treatment. You should also adhere to any employer or local guidelines on gaining consent in practice for treatment.

Using a patient-centred approach to prescribing, you should be aware of any social, religious or cultural factors that may impact on a patient's choice of treatment that may affect your prescribing decisions. For example, vegetarians will not want gelatine-based capsules.

As discussed earlier, when considering off label prescribing, you must clearly explain to the patient if you are prescribing outside of the marketing authorisation. If you are prescribing a medication in a way that is not specified on the Summary of Product Characteristics or manufacturer's data sheets, then this is off licence/off label prescribing and the patient needs to be fully informed in order to give their consent to treatment. The patient has a right to refuse any treatment you may wish to prescribe for them; however, if they do, you need to explain the risks and potential outcomes of this decision so that they are fully informed.

Breach of Duty of Care

As a paramedic prescriber, you have a duty of care to your patients. A duty of care is to provide the best care based on the best evidence available in a timely and professional way, causing no harm. Once a duty of care has been established, it needs to be demonstrated that the practitioner caused a breach of duty of care. The actions and/ or omissions of the practitioner will need to be explored to ascertain if they reached the accepted level of competence. In order for this to occur, the practitioner's actions are judged by the standards of their peers in the same role. This is the legal standing in the UK decided following the landmark case *Bolam v Friern Hospital Management Committee* (1957).

Negligence

Negligence is the neglect of care of a patient. Negligence in prescribing practice is the failing to provide a duty of care, failing to exercise reasonable care and that the breach of duty resulted in poor or adverse outcomes for the patient.

Failing to provide adequate information on a medicine you prescribe or failing to undertake a through and holistic patient assessment as part of your consultation could result in negligence of your patient. It is negligent in law to fail to communicate appropriately (Dimond, 2015). You will need to ensure that not only do you communicate all the required information to the patient, but that your record keeping reflects this discussion. Prescribing is a complex and potentially risky activity. You need to ensure that you are prescribing within your scope of prescribing practice, that you are clinically competent, skilled and knowledgeable to do so, and that your prescribing decision is based on the best available evidence and made in partnership with your patient.

Ethical Considerations

In considering an ethical approach to prescribing practice, it is essential to consider the ethical principles of Beauchamp and Childress (2013). There are other models for ethical practice that can be accessed by paramedic prescribers for consideration.

Autonomy

Autonomy is to respect the patient's right to choose. There is a focus in contemporary healthcare practice to facilitate a patient-centred shared decision-making approach to ensure that the patient's voice is heard and that the patient is able to make informed decisions about their care. It is essential, therefore, that this is incorporated into prescribing consultations and decision making. As a paramedic prescriber, you will need to respect the decisions of your patients to refuse or decline treatment that you would like to initiate, or to choose a different course of action. It is essential that you ensure that the patient has the information on which to make an informed decision and is aware of the potential outcomes should they not take your advice. You will also need to ensure that this information is clearly documented in the patient notes. The use of Patient Information Sheets, available with medicines, may help patients reach an informed decision on the proposed course of action.

Non-maleficence

This is the principle that outlines the concept to 'do no harm'. As a paramedic prescriber, you will consider any adverse effects that the medicine you wish to prescribe may have and to fully inform the patient of these. In a patient-centred and shared decision-making approach, you will need to weigh up the risk-benefit ratio of commencing a medication with potential adverse effects, using your expertise and patient choice. You will also have the ethical duty to consider any potential interactions that adding a new medication to the patient's medication regime may have.

Beneficence

This is the ethical principle of 'doing good' and is central of the professional paramedic role and healthcare practice. In undertaking this process, you will be ensuring that you are seeking out the best available prescribing option for your patient as an individual. This will be based on a person-centred holistic assessment and the best available evidence. It is imperative to ensure a patient centred approach to this ethical principle so that you are not paternalistic in your prescribing practice but are able to work in partnership with your patients, ensuring autonomy and shared decision making.

Justice

This is the ethical principle of 'fairness', although the breadth of justice in healthcare is much wider than this. In fiscal healthcare markets it is essential as a prescriber that paramedics consider the cost implications of individual prescribing decisions and the wider cost of prescribing. This can include considering prescribing within formularies, contributing to the development of formularies and considering if medicine use is effective for the patients you care for. It is important to remember that is considering justice in contemporary health care that this can be distributive justice. This includes ensuring that your prescribing practice should be cost effective so that resources are sustainable. The overriding principle being that resources should be available to all on point of need. For example, you may advise a patient to purchase paracetamol over the counter rather than prescribe it, as this is a more cost-effective and sustainable option.

Good Practice Considerations

It is essential to consider 'good practice' elements of prescribing practice when considering the legal and ethical implications of practice.

You must never prescribe for yourself. This would not be a legal prescription. You should be registered with your own medical practitioner in order to seek treatment for yourself.

Best practice indicates that you should never prescribe for family or for people close to you. The people you prescribe for should be under your care in a professional context as patients.

Only in exceptional circumstances may you prescribe for family, friends or colleagues. The College of Paramedics (2018b) identifies these circumstances as:

♦ when no other prescriber is available to assess the clinical condition and to delay prescribing would put their life of health at risk or cause intolerable pain
♦ the treatment is immediately necessary to save life, avoid serious deterioration in the patient's health or wellbeing or alleviate otherwise uncontrollable pain.

If this were to happen in practice and there was any subsequent questioning of your actions or any adverse outcomes experienced by the patient, then you would have to justify your actions to your employer, the HCPC and potentially in court. This could jeopardise your prescribing qualification and your professional registration, and is therefore best avoided.

Your choice of treatment should be based on the best available evidence and reached in agreement with your patient. As part of their promotional activities, pharmaceutical company drug representatives may provide inexpensive gifts such as pens. Personal gifts that influence prescribing practice are not permitted and it is specified in the Human Medicines Regulations (2012) by law that a prescriber may not solicit or accept a gift, advantage, benefit or hospitality that could influence your prescribing decisions.

Record Keeping

Prescribing activity should occur at the time of the consultation or contact with the patient to ensure it is contemporary and reflective of the actual events. Only in exceptional circumstances should the documentation occur after the prescribing event and this should never exceed 24 hours (College of Paramedics, 2018a).

Your prescribing record should evidence that you have communicated the prescribing activity and decision with the patient's primary healthcare practitioner, such as their GP. For inpatient care, this could be in the form of a discharge letter.

Prescribing for Children

Prescribing for children comes with its own risks. Medicines are more potent in use for children and therefore carry a higher risk of adverse outcomes, as responses to medicines may be different. You should only prescribe for children if this is within your scope of prescribing practice and you are clinically competent, experienced, skilled and knowledgeable to do so. You should also only prescribe for children with your employer's support and with indemnity insurance. You should refer to national and local policy guidance and the BNF for children before prescribing for children.

Prescribing in Pregnancy

Prescribing in pregnancy and for breastfeeding women carries increased risk. This is because of the risk of medicines reaching the baby and having a toxic effect. You should only prescribe in pregnancy and for breastfeeding women if this is within your scope of prescribing practice and you are clinically competent, experienced, skilled and knowledgeable to do so. You should also only prescribe for children with your employer's support and with indemnity insurance. It is important to remember that you are not prescribing in isolation and that there are many sources of support available to you when you are making prescribing decisions in complex areas such as pregnancy. You can call on colleagues in specialist areas to advise you, such as obstetrics, and colleagues in pharmacy will also support you. Your BNF will also offer a comprehensive guide. It is important to assess and consider the risk-benefit ratio of a prescribing decision in your practice, i.e. is it safer to prescribe or not prescribe?

However, you must remember that you are accountable for all your decisions and omissions, and therefore if you are unsure, or if this is outside of your prescribing practice you should refer on, document, and be able to justify your actions.

Prescribing and Dispensing, Prescribing and Administration

Except in very exceptional circumstances, there should always be a separation of the prescribing of and the dispensing or administration of medicines. If in exceptional circumstances a paramedic prescriber is prescribing and dispensing, then a second competent person should be involved in the checking process. Should this happen, the clear arrangements need to be in place to ensure patient and prescriber safety, and robust audit processes need to be in place.

This is reflective of the prescribing and administration of medicines. This should only happen in exceptional circumstances and in the best interests of the patient, a second person should check the medicine before administration to verify it is correct.

Controlled Drugs

Subject to changes to the Misuse of Drugs Act (1971), paramedic independent prescribers will be able to prescribe from a list of controlled drugs that are deemed necessary to ensure that patients can access optimal treatment in a timely manner. The controlled drugs that independent paramedic prescribers will be able to prescribe will reflect the conditions of patients most often seen by paramedics in practice and will follow best practice and evidence-based guidance (College of Paramedics, 2018a).

Caution must be employed when prescribing controlled drugs as these can cause dependence in some patients. You must consider prescribing controlled drugs with caution as a paramedic prescriber, and this prescribing activity should not be taken in isolation. You must follow local policy and guidance in the prescribing of controlled drugs.

As an independent prescriber, you must ensure that the prescription for controlled drugs is on the correct form. You may also instruct another person to administer controlled drugs, in the form of an authorisation chart, for example.

You must prescribe controlled drugs at the time of need and must not prescribe more than what is needed for the immediate supply, and never more than a 30-day supply.

You can use computer-generated prescriptions for controlled drugs as long as there is an audit trail of your prescriptions. Your signature must be handwritten. Best practice is not to use sticky labels on prescriptions for controlled drugs.

You must not prescribe controlled drugs for yourself or for anyone close to you, such as friend, family member, or anyone who is known to you socially, or on balance may be able to exert pressure on you to prescribe.

NICE offers evidence-based guidelines on the safe use and management of controlled drugs; there is also useful comprehensive information on the BNF to assist prescribers.

Evidence-Based Prescribing

The act of prescribing is only one part of the decision-making process. Evidence-based prescribing is an approach to decision making, considering and applying the best available evidence in the treatment of your patients (Courtenay and Griffiths 2010). When drawing on evidence, paramedic prescribers should source national primary evidence in the first instance. If this is not available, then you can turn to local protocols or evidence for prescribing (College of Paramedics, 2018a). This will be relative to the context in which your patient is presenting, as evidence-based practice differs from primary to secondary care. For example, an elderly patient presenting with a cough and comorbidities may receive first line antibiotics in primary care, however in hospital they may receive a chest x-ray and blood testing.

Paramedic prescribers need to ensure that their practice is evidence-based, and need to be aware of the current evidence supporting the use of each medicine within your scope of prescribing practice. You should only prescribe according to the best available evidence to ensure efficacy of treatment and in order to minimise risk, adverse drug reactions and interactions, and to ensure that the most appropriate medicine is chosen (College of Paramedics, 2018a).

As discussed previously in this chapter, prescribing needs to be appropriate as well as evidence-based, and patients must be involved in the prescribing decision and be able to make informed choices regarding their choices, where possible. This may not be possible where a patient lacks capacity to make decisions. To ensure safe and effective evidence-based prescribing, the College of Paramedics (2018a) has developed a 'must do' list, which is detailed in **Box 2.4**.

Box 2.4 – Paramedic prescribers 'must do' list

♦ Be familiar with national sources of evidence. For example: National Institute for Health and Care Excellence (NICE), British Thoracic Society (BTS), Scottish Intercollegiate Guidelines Network (SIGN).
♦ Be familiar with the national sources of evidence for the condition you are treating, what should and should not be used, and the hierarchy of medicine use. NICE and the BNF can provide valuable information sources.
♦ Take an appropriate holistic assessment of the patient.
♦ Take into account the patient's wishes and choices.
♦ Prescribe the appropriate dose for the patient's age, weight, height and medical history.
♦ Prescribe the correct duration and frequency of the medicine.

(College of Paramedics, 2018)

Conclusion

This chapter has highlighted how the legal and ethical principles you apply in your practice can be adapted to prescribing practice by paramedics. Ensuring that you apply these principles will promote safe and effective decision making in prescribing practice. A key factor is to ensure that you involve the patient in the prescribing decision-making process, and take care to make contemporaneous and detailed records that reflect the consultation and identify the rationale of the prescribing decision. The patient's perspective should also be included in your documentation.

Another key consideration is to ensure that you prescribe in your scope of prescribing practice and refer on when you feel that there is a prescribing decision to be made outside of your scope of prescribing practice or competence. You must always have assessed the patient you are prescribing for and must never prescribe in order to fill a deficit in the availability of others' ability to prescribe in practice, for example if a lack of resourcing is available.

Always ensure an evidence-based approach to your prescribing practice, based on the most recent and available national evidence, and be prepared to justify your prescribing decision to others based on this.

Key Points of This Chapter

♦ There is clear guidance provided by the College of Paramedics, which has a foundation in the legal system surrounding prescribing.
♦ Paramedic prescribers also need to be cognisant of the ethical considerations when prescribing.
♦ There are many factors that require the consideration of the paramedic prescriber, but ultimately you must only prescribe in the areas in which you are knowledgeable and skilled to do so safely.

References

Beauchamp, T.L. and Childress, J.F. (2013). *Principles of Biomedical Ethics*, 7th ed. New York: Oxford University Press.

British National Formulary (BNF) (2017). *The British National Formulary 74, September 2017–March 2018*. London: The BMJ Group.

College of Paramedics (2015). *Paramedic Career Framework*. Bridgwater: College of Paramedics.

College of Paramedics (2018a). *Practice Guidance for Paramedic Independent and Supplementary Prescribers*. Bridgwater: College of Paramedics.

College of Paramedics (2018b). *Improving Patients' Access to Medicines: A guide to implementing paramedic prescribing with the NHS in the UK*. Bridgwater: College of Paramedics.

Courtenay, M. and Griffiths, M. (2010). *Independent and Supplementary Prescribing: An essential guide*. Cambridge: Cambridge University Press.

Department of Health (1989). *Report for the Advisory Group on Nurse Prescribing (Crown Report)*. London: Department of Health.

Dimond, B. (2015). *Legal Aspects of Nursing*. 7th ed. London: Pearson.

England, E. (2016). Paramedics and medicines: legal considerations. *Journal of Paramedic Practice*, 8(8): 408–15.

Health Care Professions Council (HCPC) (2013). *Standards for Prescribing*. London: HCPC.

Health Care Professions Council (HCPC) (2018). *Medicines and Prescribing*. Available at: http://www.hcpc-uk.co.uk/aboutregistration/medicinesandprescribing [last accessed 8 July 2018].

Health Education England (2016). *Advanced Clinical Practice*. London: Health Education England.

HM Government (1968). *Medicines Act*. London: The Stationery Office.

HM Government (1971). *Misuse of Drugs Act*. London: The Stationery Office.

HM Government (2012). *Humans Medicines Regulations*. London: The Stationery Office.

NHS Education for Scotland (2016). *Advanced Nursing Practice Service Needs Analysis Tool*. Scotland: NHS.

NHS Education for Scotland (Nursing, Midwifery and Allied Health Professions). (2018) *Out of Hours Unscheduled Care: Advanced Clinical Practice Portfolio*. Available at: https://www.nes.scot.nhs.uk/media/463876/ooh_advanced_clinical_practice_portfolio.pdf [last accessed 10 August 2018].

NHS Wales. National Leadership and Innovation Agency for Healthcare (2018). *Framework for Advancing Nursing, Midwifery and Allied Health Professional Practice in Wales*. Available at: http://www.nwssp.wales.nhs.uk/sitesplus/documents/1178/NLIAH%20Advanced%20Practice%20Framework.pdf [last accessed 10 August 2018].

Chapter 3
Assessing Health: History Taking and Consultation

Hannah Morris

In This Chapter

- Introduction
- Health assessment
- Assessment and consultation
- Consultation models
- Wider determinants of health
- Age, sex and constitutional factors
- Individual lifestyle factors
- Social and community networks
- General socio-economic, cultural and environmental conditions
- 'Must dos' for safe prescribing
- Conclusion
- Key points of this chapter
- References

Introduction

This chapter aims to provide a context for health assessment for prescribing practice for paramedics. This will include concepts of history taking and consultation styles for prescribing practice. As an experienced and advanced paramedic, you will have a wealth of personal experience in your area of practice. The assessment and consultation skills learnt as part of your professional registration are well practised and you are an expert in your field of paramedic practice; however, your skills may need to be refined as you take on the role of an independent prescriber.

For the majority of new independent prescribers, across the disciplines, the focus of health assessment, history taking and consultation skills will be on analysing your current framework of assessment and consultation, and identifying adaptations you may need to make to support your prescribing decisions.

Health Assessment

The purpose of any health assessment is to gather a history. As part of this history, you may undertake your primary and secondary survey (Blaber and Harris, 2016). The health assessment process is an opportunity for the patient–practitioner relationship to develop and deepen.

Intrinsic to health assessment in a prescribing context is the need to have an outcome of a diagnosis or differential diagnoses, made through clinical reasoning of the findings of the assessment processes. As you will be well aware, the key to making an accurate diagnosis on which to base your prescribing decision is eliciting a good history through the processes of primary and secondary survey (Blaber and Harris, 2016).

Clinical reasoning is the identification of problems or symptoms that the patient 'presents' with. This will include the identification of any abnormalities in the findings of any examinations undertaken. The skilled practitioner will then link the findings to the underlying pathophysiology in order to establish a set of explanations of causes for such abnormalities. Through this process of hypothetical deductive reasoning (Elsien and Scharz, 2002), the skilled paramedic can create a hypothesis to form a set of differential diagnoses for interpretation. In considering the 'differentials', a working diagnosis can then be formed by reviewing findings with the available evidence base. It is the skilled and experienced clinician who is able to direct a sensitive and nuanced history through relevant questioning in order to elicit an accurate history on which to base their prescribing decisions.

As clinical reasoning and clinical decision making is complex and multi-faceted in paramedic practice, it will be discussed in more depth in **Chapter 5**.

There are a number of factors that support the health assessment and clinical reasoning in paramedic practice. These include:

♦ the patient's story
♦ multi-morbidity
♦ medication and drug history
♦ polypharmacy
♦ altered pathophysiology
♦ the wider determinants of health.

These will be well known to you; however, it is worth revisiting what resources are available to you in formulating a hypothesis and diagnosis in prescribing practice; as we have already identified, the key to making an accurate diagnosis is through an accurate and thorough assessment and history.

Obviously the patient's story will inform your clinical reasoning, should they be able or willing to tell you what the problem is. This is not always the case and prescribers have to rely on other sources of information from third parties, such as families or friends when available, whilst considering the legal and ethical implications of this. The examinations and investigations you choose to carry out in your secondary survey based on your primary survey findings will help build up a picture of what is occurring with the pathophysiology. For example, if your patient presents with increased dyspnoea and an audible wheeze, then investigation and examination related to respiratory assessment will give a wider picture of what may be occurring.

Assessment and Consultation

Using a primary survey, you will elicit any life-threatening issues and risk manage any prescribing situation that you encounter, whereas a secondary survey should provide an opportunity to undertake a focused history and physical examination to identify any problems (Blaber and Harris, 2016).

Through a secondary survey, you will be well versed in taking a history through eliciting a presenting complaint, past medical history, drug and medical history, and undertaking a review of the body systems (Blaber and Harris, 2016). Through this process, you may use frameworks such as SOCRATES to assess pain (AACE 2013).

Case Study 3.1

You are a paramedic prescriber working in the minor injuries department of a small cottage hospital. Your next patient is a six-year-old girl with a rash on her face; she has been bought in by her mum along with her younger sister after advice from the school. Your patient is very timid and reluctant to talk to you as she is frightened. Her last experience of attending hospital, due to a broken arm, meant that she had to stay in overnight. This is not something she would like to do again. You want to make this a positive experience.

HPC 4/7 history of red lesions that are beginning to weep

PMH: # L wrist

Allergies: none

DH: none

SH: lives with mum and sister

SE: no systemic signs of illness

OE: HR 116 beats per minute (bpm)

    Blood glucose 4.8 mmols

    RR 22 breaths per minute (bpm)

    Temp 36.7 °C

IMP: impetigo

Plan: hygiene advice – wash affected areas with soapy water, wash hands after touching the area, avoid scratching, do not share towels or face cloths.

Keep off school until the lesions have dried or scabbed over, as mum reports going to school and being teased about her facial rash is causing anxiety for her daughter.

Topical antibiotics: fusidic acid QDS 1/52.

Check patient's mother and sister for signs of impetigo.

For prescribing practice, it is essential that you are able to draw on the assessment skills that you have and incorporate a prescribing perspective in doing so to adopt a consultation approach. By doing this, you will be able to facilitate a patient-centred and shared decision-making approach to your prescribing practice. Each consultation for prescribing will take an individual stance or approach depending on the patient, the context and the presenting complaint (see **Case Study 3.1**). Each consultation should follow the same principles:

♦ patient-centred
♦ professional
♦ evidence-informed
♦ shared decision making.

Case Study 3.1 highlights the importance of the care being delivered by the practitioner who makes the initial diagnosis. This avoids undue distress and frustration caused by multiple practitioners carrying out the same assessment to enable them to prescribe. The case study demonstrates the effectiveness of prescribing, enabling the paramedic to make patient encounters truly patient-centred, professional and evidence-based. In this case the shared decision making was between the paramedic and the patient's mother.

Consultation Models

There are a plethora of consultation models available for use for prescribing practice that assist the practitioner in undertaking a structured consultation, drawing on their communication skills and experience whilst developing prescribing practice. Not all available models of consultation can be discussed here; however, a few are outlined to a basis for consulting with patients, with recommendations for paramedic prescribing practice.

The Pendleton et al. (1984) model offers a patient-centred approach to a prescribing consultation in discussing their ideas, concerns and expectations (ICE). This includes:

1. defining the reason for attending
2. consider other problems
3. with the patient, choose an appropriate plan
4. achieve a shared understanding with the patient
5. involve the patient with managing the plan
6. use time and resources effectively
7. establish and maintain a relationship.

Neighbour (1987) outlines similar contexts in his model, building on that of Pendleton et al. (1984), where he includes the acknowledgement that intentions and plans of the prescribing consultation may not always turn out as expected. He also incorporates some reflective practice to prescribing in his model:

♦ connecting (relationship building)
♦ summarising (reaching a shared understanding, considering ICE)
♦ handing over (shared decision making in the prescribing plan)

- safety netting (what to do if things don't go to plan)
- housekeeping (reflective practice).

A commonly used and well-known model of consultation is the Calgary-Cambridge model (Silverman et al., 1998):

- initiating the session
- gathering information
- building a relationship
- explanation and planning
- closing the session.

This model includes shared decision making and a patient-centred focus though the patient setting the agenda without relinquishing all of the decision making by the paramedic prescriber. It offers structure and direction; however, it does not consider reflection as part of prescribing practice or the wider governance and strategic perspectives of paramedic prescribing practice.

The National Prescribing Centre (1999) formulated a framework to guide the seven principles of safe prescribing practice to assist in decision making (see **Figure 3.1**), which has been used by nurse independent prescribers as a consultation and step-by-step approach to prescribing practice since they have been able to undertake prescribing in practice.

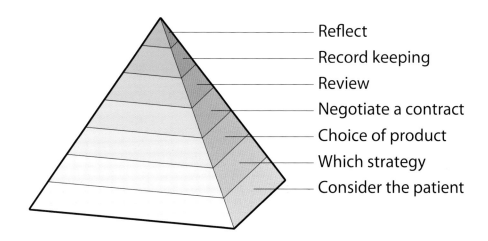

Reflect
Record keeping
Review
Negotiate a contract
Choice of product
Which strategy
Consider the patient

Figure 3.1 – The prescribing pyramid

Source: National Prescribing Centre (1999). *Nurse Prescribing Bulletin.* Signposts for prescribing nurses – general principles of good prescribing. London: NPC

Consideration of the Patient

- Who is the patient?
- Is it appropriate for you to prescriber for them within your scope of prescribing practice?
- What is the presenting complaint?
- How long has it been going on?
- Has anything been tried already?
- Is the patient taking any other medication that may affect your decision?

Which Strategy?

- Consider if there is a working diagnosis that has been established.
- Is a referral on to another healthcare professional/prescriber indicated?
- Is a prescription needed?
- Is patient expectation a factor?
- What treatment options are available?

It is important to remember that a prescription should only be issued if there is a genuine need. A prescription should only be issued if on balance this is the best option for the patient at the time of presentation and within the context of this presentation.

Considering the Product

The National Prescribing Centre (NPC) (1999) offers the mnemonic EASE to assist in deciding how to select a product to prescribe:

- E: how **E**ffective is the product?
- A: is it **A**ppropriate for this person?
- S: how **S**afe is it?
- E: is the prescription cost **E**ffective?

Negotiate a Contract

- Has shared decision making taken place?
- Does the patient know how to take this medication correctly and safely?
- What safety netting has taken place, do they know what to do and who to contact if something goes wrong?

Review the Patient

- Consider what follow-up is needed.
- Consider repeat prescribing and your prescribing role and scope of prescribing practice.

Record Keeping

♦ Consider the College of Paramedics and the HCPC and your employer's requirements for safe and effective contemporaneous record keeping.
♦ Consider that there needs to be a clear audit trial to inform further prescribing decision making.

Reflection

♦ Reflective practice improves prescribing practice.
♦ Consider what has gone well as well as what has not gone so well.
♦ Action plan for your future prescribing practice.
♦ What learning and development needs have been identified?
♦ What can others learn from this?
♦ Who do you need to support you?

The *Competency Framework for All Prescribers* (Royal Pharmaceutical Society (RPS), 2016) (**Figure 3.2**) offers a structured patient-centred consultation framework specifically for prescribing practitioners to use, incorporating consideration of prescribing governance issues. It is at this time a consultation model.

The model (RPS, 2016) also incorporates the competencies required for all prescribers to achieve safe and effective patient-centred prescribing. It is these competencies that you will need to demonstrate you have achieved when undertaking the independent prescribing course. The College of Paramedics expects all prescribing paramedic members to be able to demonstrate how they meet this competency framework (College of Paramedics, 2018). Therefore, due to the specific prescribing nature of this consultation framework and its mapping to the competencies required for all prescribers, it is highly recommended that this is the consultation framework that is adopted by paramedics undertaking prescribing practice.

The consultation model detailed in **Figure 3.2** can be used in conjunction with the prescribing pyramid's seven principles (**Figure 3.1**) to safe prescribing (NPC, 1999) as your prescribing experience develops, as this will encourage reflective prescribing practice.

Turn to **Chapter 10** for more detail on reflective practice.

It is important in prescribing practice to refer to your practice experience in making prescribing decisions. As paramedics, you will have gained a wide level of experience and knowledge in your area of expertise and this will form the basis of your clinical reasoning and decision making. You will pick up cues from your patients about what they are experiencing through the language that is used, both verbally and non-verbally, and you will be able to interpret this by drawing on your experience and

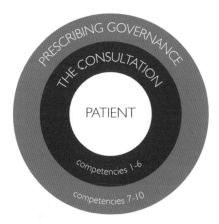

THE CONSULTATION	PRESCRIBING GOVERNANCE
1. Assess the patient	7. Prescribe safely
2. Consider the options	8. Prescribe professionally
3. Reach a shared decision	9. Improve prescribing practice
4. Prescribe	10. Prescribe as part of a team
5. Provide information	
6. Monitor and review	

Figure 3.2 – The Competency Framework for All Prescribers model

Source: Royal Pharmaceutical Society (2016). *The Competency Framework for All Prescribers*. London: Royal Pharmaceutical Society.

intuition. I use the word 'intuition' as a nurse, and there has long been a debate about the use of intuition in nursing practice. What I mean to refer to is 'how you know things' in practice and this relates to paramedic practice too. This can be about cue recognition, from what you may have seen or heard in your experience; it can also relate to the assimilation of theoretical knowledge from the classroom into practice situations. The key here is not to use 'intuition' or whatever way of describing 'what you know you know' in prescribing practice in isolation, but to utilise your experience concurrently with your experience, the clinical presentation and assessment findings, and the evidence base available to you.

Turn to **Chapter 5** where clinical decision making is explained further.

Wider Determinants of Health

A key element of health assessment on which to base safe and effective prescribing decisions is the consideration of the holistic need of patients and the influences on the health of the individual. As prescribers, we need to consider the wider determinants of health. Dahlgren and Whitehead (1991) formulated the concept of the wider determinants of health when looking at strategies to promote social equity in health. The model has utility today in considering influences on health and how this may affect your prescribing decision making in practice; see **Figure 3.3**.

Think about...

It is useful to think about how these wider determinants of health may influence your prescribing decisions in paramedic prescribing practice.

Looking at **Figure 3.3**, consider how each determinant may have an influence on your decision making as an independent prescriber.

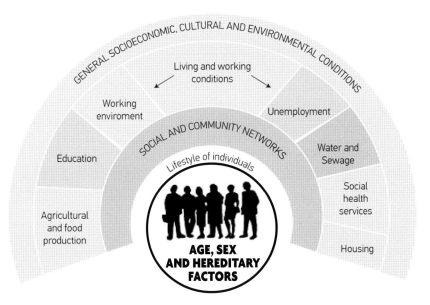

Figure 3.3 – Wider determinants of health

Source: Dahlgren, G. and Whitehead, M. (1991). *Policies and Strategies to Promote Social Equity in Health.* Stockholm: Institute of Future Studies.

Age, Sex and Constitutional Factors

Considering age, sex and constitutional factors at the centre of the rainbow (see **Figure 3.3**), we can identify that these factors have an impact on our health. For example, as we age, we become less well and more prone to disease, and our gender will pre-dispose us to certain health and disease risk factors. When considering prescribing decisions, you will need to consider a patient's age and gender.

Ageing and Multi-morbidity

As people age, they are more likely to develop co-morbidities complicating the course of intervention and treatment that can be offered; this will be a major consideration in your prescribing decision making. The presence of two or more long-term conditions is now considered multi-morbidity; this is associated with a poorer quality of life and a greater use of health resources, such as medicines and appointments.

Prescribing decisions in multi-morbidity need to be patient-centred. Special attention should be paid to patient choice and quality of life outcomes. When considering prescribing in multiple pathologies, it is advisable to consider the evidence available for single disease pathology and discuss this with the patient. Evidence sources such as NICE treatment guidelines are a valuable resource, but it must be remembered in prescribing practice that these evidence sources are compiled from research into people experiencing single disease pathology. It is essential to remember that the patient with multiple long-term disease pathology is likely to be an expert in their health, and their opinion should be sought and included in any decision.

In prescribing for symptom relief in multi-pathology, it is essential to consider any treatment for its effectiveness and its evidence base for use. This needs to include the stopping and reducing of medicines and monitoring the effects. Non-pharmacological interventions for symptom relief should also be considered in multi-pathology to reduce the treatment burden. In considering prescribing for predicted risk of future disease is a special consideration in multi-pathology as it is not always advisable to increase the medication and treatment burden to those with multiple chronic health needs (BNF, 2017).

Turn to **Chapter 2** for more information on evidence-based practice.

Polypharmacy

Initiating one medication for one complaint will have a potentially huge impact on another condition. Concurrent with multiple co-morbidities in age, people will inadvertently have multiple medications to treat and manage these conditions, which will result in polypharmacy.

Again, the more medications people take, the more problems they are likely to experience due to their ability to manage multiple medicines effectively, they may be more likely to experience interactions and adverse effects from polypharmacy. In addition, as people age, they will be more likely to have had a previous experience of an adverse drug reaction, reducing the choice of treatments that you have to consider when you prescribe.

De-prescribing

De-prescribing is the process of reducing or discontinuing medications or dose by a prescriber to manage polypharmacy (BNF, 2017). Due to the issues outlined above, de-prescribing should be part of your routine clinical prescribing assessment strategy, as **Case Study 3.2** highlights. Any de-prescribing decisions should be undertaken in partnership with patients in a shared decision-making approach. This facilitates a person-centred approach to prescribing practice, but also encourages the taking of medicines to their best effects with the least likely opportunity of an unwanted outcome.

Case Study 3.2 highlights the importance of taking a thorough history and reviewing all medications prescribed, whether they be long-standing prescriptions or additional medications for short-term use. Patients will sometimes only mention medications that they take regularly over a long period of time.

Altered Pathology in Ageing

Age also brings with it altered pathology and end organ failure. Of particular concern in prescribing practice is liver and renal disease due to pharmacokinetics.

Liver Disease

Liver disease can alter the response of drugs and, as such, prescribing in all patients with liver disease should be kept to a minimum. Problems particularly occur in patients experiencing jaundice, encephalopathy and ascites. Metabolism by the liver is a route of elimination for many drugs; however, liver disease has to be quite severe to alter the metabolism of drugs. Routine liver function tests are a not a reliable source of estimating the liver's capacity to metabolise drugs and therefore should not be routinely undertaken. Similarly, it is not possible to ascertain how likely an extent individual may metabolise a drug. Therefore, prescribing for liver disease should be undertaken with extreme caution and by prescribing practitioners working in the speciality of hepatic care (BNF, 2017).

Other important points to note in liver disease when making prescribing decisions and reviewing medications include the following:

♦ Reduced clotting increases the sensitivity to oral coagulants such as warfarin from a prolonged prothrombin time, caused by reduced hepatic synthesis of blood clotting.

Case Study 3.2

You are working as a paramedic on an ambulance and you are called to a 46-year-old female with mild difficulty in breathing. Cause?

HPC: two-hour history of wheezing and mild shortness of breath. No aggravating or relieving factors

PMH: 1/7 non-bony shoulder injury, seen in the ED and prescribed diclofenac

Nasal polyps

No previous episodes of breathing problems

Allergies: none known

DH: Diclofenac 5/7

SH: lives with partner

SE: no chest pain, no chest tightness, no cyanosis, no oedema, no pursing of lips, able to continue activities of daily living, no cough, no sore throat

OE: respiratory exam – no consolidation

bilateral pan expiratory wheeze

HR 96 beats per minute (bpm)

BP 125/65 mmHg

Blood glucose 4.8 mmols

RR 24 breaths per minute (bpm)

Temp 36.8°C

SpO$_2$ 96%

IMP: allergic reaction caused by non-steroidal anti-inflammatory drugs (NSAIDs)

Plan: treat the wheeze following asthma guidelines, ensuring an ABC approach.

De-prescribe NSAIDs.

Consider prescribing COX-2 inhibitor.

Ensure advice is given to patient about the type of allergy and not to take medication containing this type of NSAID in the future.

Contact patient's GP.

- Reduced protein binding in hypoproteinaemia in severe liver disease can cause toxicity of highly protein bound drugs such as phenytoin.
- Oedema and ascites can be exacerbated by drugs that cause fluid retention such as NSAIDs and corticosteroids.
- In severe liver disease, some drugs can impair brain function and cause hepatic encephalopathy. Sedatives, opioids and diuretics should be avoided, as should any drug that causes a risk of constipation (BNF, 2017).

Renal Disease

Prescribing in renal disease should also be undertaken with caution. However, in renal disease, even if suspected due to the clinical picture, then renal function should be checked before prescribing any medication that may require drug modification in renal disease.

The main issues encountered in renal disease and impaired renal function can cause problems for many reasons. These include the following:

- Reduced excretion by the kidneys may cause toxicity of the drug.
- Sensitivity to some drugs can be increased in renal disease, even if there is no impairment to an individual's elimination of the drug.
- Some drugs can be ineffective when there is a reduction in renal function.
- People who experience renal disease and poor renal function may not be able to tolerate the side-effects of some medications (BNF, 2017).

Many of these problems can be minimised through effective prescribing of reduced doses or the replacement of drugs with different medicines. Patient-centred prescribing is of value; listening to the patient and their experiences of the issues encountered and the side-effects of their medications will lead to safe and effective prescribing practice in renal disease, in a patient-centred approach. Patients who experience renal disease and therefore require special consideration in prescribing practice are likely to require follow up and review.

Turn to **Chapter 9**, where patient factors and prescribing prescribing is discussed in more depth.

Individual Lifestyle Factors

Each individual's choice of lifestyle and associated lifestyle factors will have an impact on the prescribing decisions you make. Lifestyle behaviours not only have an impact on health and health outcomes, but also on the medications and options you have to prescribe.

You will have considered a social or family history as part of your secondary survey; however, for prescribing in paramedic practice, you will also need to consider a wider perspective on lifestyle factors, as this is a critical aspect on which to make your prescribing decisions. All illness treatment and interventions should be seen in the context of the individual and should include consideration of beliefs, personality and spirituality. Occupation, environment, interests and behaviours, such as smoking and alcohol consumption, have a profound impact on health and disease.

Similar to eliciting a presenting complaint as part of your secondary survey, there are mnemonics for social assessment and history taking that need to be considered for safe and effective holistic person-centred decision making in prescribing practice. These can be seen in **Box 3.1**.

Box 3.1 – Mnemonics for social assessment

SAFE   S- Smoking
         A-Alcohol
         F- Food
         E- Exercise

HELP   H- Housing
         E- Employment
         L- Living/dependants
         P- Pets

HAT   H- Hobbies
         A- Activities
         T- Travel

Source: D. Nuttall and J. Rutt-Howland (2011). *The Textbook of Non-Medical Prescribing*, Wiley-Blackwell.

Smoking

Smoking is a lifestyle choice with the now well-known risks to poor health outcomes as it is of the most common causes of lung disease and the main cause of chronic obstructive pulmonary disease (COPD). As such, smoking may often be hidden from prescribing practitioners by patients, carers and families due to the stigma that has become associated with it. Assessing smoking-related activity is part of any assessment. For example, evidence of smoking, or smoking in the home will help inform your clinical diagnosis and affect the decision to prescribe oxygen due to the associated risk of fire. Similarly, smoking needs to be considered in patients with long-term conditions. Not only does smoking increase the severity of dyspnoea and disease progression in pathologies such as heart failure and COPD, it is an associated cardiovascular risk in type 2 diabetes (Meerabeau and Wright, 2011) and can also worsen the symptoms of multiple sclerosis (Wingerchuk, 2012). Such issues may affect your prescribing decision making in terms of what medication and titration you may have to consider for individual patients when prescribing for smokers in these pathologies. Likewise, it is essential to consider if the drug you wish to prescribe is affected by smoking. For example, clozapine used for psychosis in Parkinson's disease may need dose adjustment should smoking be started or stopped during treatment (BNF, 2017).

Alcohol

Alcohol misuse is a huge public health issue in the UK. Alcohol misuse in the elderly population is increasing (Holley-Moore and Beach, 2016) and, as such, has risk factors for prescribing practice. Again, alcohol consumption may be hidden from prescribing practitioners due to the social stigma it carries and if it is reported in a secondary survey, it may be difficult to ascertain an accurate picture of consumption and frequency. Alcohol intake needs to be considered in prescribing practice as it has many risk factors when taken concomitant with certain medications and can cause hepatotoxicity; caution and consideration is required in the prescribing decision-making process.

Due to its anticoagulant affect, alcohol needs to be considered when prescribing drugs with the same properties, such as aspirin and warfarin, as excessive anticoagulation can occur, resulting in a risk of bleeding. Likewise, alcohol use has a gastric risk and the prescribing of gastric irritants such as NSAIDs should be done with caution, even with a proton pump inhibitor.

Alcohol use in the elderly can increase the risk of falls; therefore, prescribing drugs that can exacerbate the risk of falling, such as diuretics and anti-hypertensives, should be givenspecial consideration and regular monitoring of the patient should occur. Undertaking a falls risk assessment is a useful resource to guide decision making in prescribing when falls are a consideration.

Alcohol also has sedative properties and therefore can exacerbate the effects of narcotics and tranquilisers, and this intensification should be avoided. Alcohol can also cause dehydration, and this can affect the therapeutic use of some medicines, as well as affecting the metabolism and elimination. Risk of dehydration should be considered in your assessment when making prescribing decisions where alcohol misuse is suspected. Alcohol can have interactions with common medications that you may wish to prescribe. For example, when prescribing antibiotics, it is essential to consider alcohol use, as not only can the consumption of alcohol reduce the therapeutic effect of some antibiotics, but it can also result in serious and life-threatening interactions with antibiotics such as metronidazole.

This is by no means an exhaustive list of issues to consider in terms of smoking and alcohol in prescribing practice as a paramedic. However, it does highlight the need to be aware of the affect and impact that these lifestyle risk factors may have on the medications that make up the scope of your prescribing practice.

Food

Dietary requirements have an influence on prescribing practice. Food may be a prescribed item itself for those with special dietary requirements, and this can be an issue when considering the cost to the patient of prescriptions. Patients may not wish to use certain medications if they contain animal products such as gelatine, or have been used in animal testing, and you may need to reconsider your decision making in a patient-centred approach.

Similarly, some drugs that you may wish to prescribe within your scope of practice may have interactions with some food sources and patient counselling will be required to ensure that the concomitant use will be avoided. Consumption of grapefruit or grapefruit juice must be avoided with some medications, such as statins, calcium channel blockers and cytotoxic drugs, as it can increase the therapeutic level of the drug, leading to toxicity and increased side-effects.

Antacids are widely used in the population for heartburn and are often not reported as drugs in a medication review, as they can be purchased over the counter. It is important to assess lifestyle factors such as diet and food intake to elicit such problems as heartburn, acid reflux and indigestion. Long-term use of antacids can cause a mild magnesium deficiency which can go undiagnosed. Magnesium is required for the absorption and usage of calcium in the bones and can be a cause factor in the increase in osteoporosis in people who use these medicines for a long time. Consideration should be given to patients who present in your prescribing practice the long-term use of antacids and proton pump inhibitors, especially women.

Exercise

Exercise is a healthy lifestyle choice and should be encouraged in a public health perspective to prescribing practice. However, it should be considered that exercise can have some implications for prescribing practice. Statins can cause reversible myositis and therefore this severe muscle pain will impact on the ability to exercise. Statin use will need to be considered in patients presenting with pain requesting analgesia for muscle pain.

Lactic acidosis is the build-up of lactic acid in the muscle tissue that results from intense exercise. Some medications cause lactic acidosis, such as metformin in Type 2 diabetes, and some HIV drugs. Metformin should not be given to diabetics with hepatic or renal disease as this increases the risk of lactic acidosis. This may have considerations for your prescribing practice if you are presented with a patient with diabetes or HIV exercising for positive health outcomes and complaining of intense muscle pain.

Housing

Housing may impact on your prescribing decisions in terms of people's ability to access medication and in the storing of medication. Elderly, frail people with mobility issues may not be able to regularly access medication and may have to rely on others for this.

This should be considered when considering your prescribing decision in terms of the amount of a medicine you wish to prescribe. Storage issues in the home may occur if there is a lack of suitable storage facilities in the home, such as refrigeration for insulin or vitamin B12. Likewise, if there is a risk of misuse of medicines due to other residents in the home and the storage of high street value drugs such as codeine, narcotics or tranquilisers, this will need to be factored into your prescribing decision.

Some presenting complaints such as recurrent chest infections may have a root cause of housing issues rather than respiratory disease, and as such are worth exploring. Poor ventilation, damp, pets and lack of heating are all factors to consider in making your prescribing decisions, especially if this occurs remotely from the patient's home.

Employment

Employment will have an impact on any social or medical prescribing you may undertake in practice. A patient's employment (or lack of) will influence their ability or willingness to engage with treatment regimens that you may wish to consider. People aiming to take medications whilst working need to consider their ability to do so prior to commencing medications. This decision making in partnership with patients will increase adherence to medication regimes and prevent waste. The working environment may not be conducive to the timing of tightly controlled regimens, such as QDS insulin whilst maintaining set teaching schedules. The environment may not lend itself well to clean or aseptic techniques, such as injectables of intravenous therapy for antibiotics required on a building site. Similarly, a lack of employment or a low income may prevent some people from wishing to engage in treatment regimes that have a cost involved. This may not be restricted to prescription costs or costs of equipment such as dressings, but may include some foodstuffs or supplements that are required to complement the prescribed drug regime. Some people without employment may be experiencing poverty and may not wish to have health practitioners in their home environment.

In terms of employment, it is also paramount to consider the wider issues of the prescribed regime you wish to put forward. This includes whether the prescribed medication will affect the patient's ability to work when this is of financial or psychological importance to them. This could include the sedative effects of a medication such as benzodiazepines and some antidepressants such as sertraline on their ability to drive or concentrate. There are legal penalties for driving or being in control of a vehicle when under the influence of controlled or prescribed drugs, so caution must be taken by the prescriber and the patient (BNF, 2017). The government provides information on its public websites on the rules and regulations regarding this. This could also include the side-effects experienced being so severe that it makes fulfilling the job role challenging. For example, severe rhinitis experienced as a side-effect of citalopram for a dentist would make their job difficult, as would requiring regular toilet breaks for a community worker or flight attendant experiencing diarrhoea from antibiotic therapy.

Again, employment will have an impact if there are other prescribed regimes for the patient's condition, that require attendance at appointments concurrent with any prescribed medication regime. This needs to be considered when making shared patient-centred prescribing decisions. For example, treating chronic or a new onset of musculoskeletal pain with analgesia may be complemented by a course of physiotherapy that the patient may find difficult to attend due to their employment pattern. This also needs to be considered in the management of depression where antidepressant medication is an adjunct to talking therapies or prescribed exercise regimes that are now seen to be the more effective course of action for such depression (Meerabeau and Wright, 2011; NICE, 2009).

Paradoxically, it also needs to be considered when making prescribing decisions if the patient you are treating is legitimising their 'sick role' in a quest for medication (Meerabeau and Wright, 2011) and to avoid employment or work. This will be elicited by the skilled practitioner as part of the health assessment process, but it is paramount to work in partnership with the patient and reach a shared prescribing decision. That is not to say that any prescriber should feel pressured into making a prescribing decision at a patient's request; if in doubt, seek support from your team, pharmacists and medical prescribers.

Living/Dependants

Living can incorporate lifestyle factors as previously discussed. This concept can also include daily routines for people experiencing and managing long-term conditions or coping with the effects of ill health. For example, a person may not wish to leave their home or socialise if they feel embarrassed or stigmatised by their long-term condition, which may impact on any prescribing intervention you make. Some people with chronic leg ulceration experience malodourous exudate and may not wish to attend clinic appointments or adhere to the prescribed treatment or exercise therapy due to this. Psoriasis may result in skin shedding in public, causing embarrassment to the sufferer, resulting in social isolation. Treatment regimes can also be part of the problem as well as the solution and must be discussed in shared decision making with the patient (Meerabeau and Wright, 2011).

Someone living with COPD or heart failure may have a specific daily routine that helps them to cope with and alleviate dyspnoea. This needs to be considered when deciding on new treatment regimes, as the person with a long-term condition is the expert in managing their health, has done so for a long time and has often maintained a pattern of living that enables their independence or optimal level of independence in coping with disease pathology (Snodden, 2009).

Considering dependants not only concerns those who have children to care for whilst requiring medication regimes, but also people who undertake care as unpaid work. This may involve looking after older people or even animals. It is important to maintain a person-centred approach to prescribing, as care of others will often take precedence over care of oneself for people who undertake caring roles (Phillips, 2006). This can impact on prescribing decisions as people may find it impossible or too much of a challenge to undertake a medication regime that interferes with their existing responsibilities, such as in their employment as already discussed. To make a patient-centred and shared decision, the areas such as unpaid care work and daily living routines need to be incorporated into the prescribing decision.

Pets

Pets are an important consideration in the social assessment process. They are often a highly valued part of people's lives and therefore must be considered in making prescribing decisions. This is not just as part of the caring role, or people seeing pets as dependants. Pets can be a contributing factor to the exacerbation of disease in illness such as asthma. Allergies to animal fur can initiate or exacerbate eczema and rhinitis. While to a practitioner, it may seem sensible to avoid such triggers, to a patient, the pet may be the one element of their lives that brings them joy and quality of life. Therefore, it is important to consider how the inclusion of pets can be facilitated in daily living whilst considering medication and social prescribing that allows the patient to live well. For example, this may include the prescription of increased inhaler therapy in asthma and social prescribing of encouraging the patient to keep the cat out of the bedroom. Alternatively, it could be the prescription of some topical steroid therapy for eczema, with regular emollient therapy and encouraging the patient to cover their arms in light cotton fabric whilst horseriding.

Hobbies and Activities

Much of what has been discussed above can also be attributed to the consideration of an individual's hobbies and activities when considering prescribing decisions. The key ethos in social assessment is considering the person as an individual, with their own life and routine, and with a role in making a shared decision about a prescribing intervention that is going to be conducive to them maintaining their chosen or set lifestyle and routine. Of course, that is not to say as a prescriber that you should not take the opportunity to provide education or health promotion where it is indicated in your prescribing consultation regarding health and lifestyle behaviours. Making Every Contact Count is a health policy strategy that utilises everyday interactions to encourage and help people make healthier choices and achieve positive long-term outcomes through behaviour change (NHS England, 2014) and this should be incorporated into prescribing consultations and prescribing practice by all prescribers.

It is also of value to consider any sporting activity that your patient may undertake as a hobby, as certain medicines that you may consider prescribing may have unwanted effects on their performance or may negatively impact on any doping testing that may be undertaken. Care is needed and a shared decision-making approach, professional athletes and sports personnel will usually be well informed about any medications that they can or cannot take. Any prescriber who colludes in the provision of drugs or treatment to enhance sporting activity may have their professional registration questioned; however, this does not preclude the intention to improve or protect health (BNF, 2017).

Travel

Travel will influence prescribing decisions in terms of whether it will be possible to incorporate a prescribing decision into travel plans. Travel history and foreign travel must also be considered as part of a full health and social assessment. Recent travel may provide an indicator as to the cause of symptoms and presenting health complaints.

The BNF offers a guide on vaccinations on travel. These guidelines change frequently and therefore the most current and up-to-date information should be sought when counselling a patient with this advice or eliciting a health history. Health information on overseas travel for professionals can be accessed at www.nathnac.org.

People travelling to the UK from abroad may have medications that do not have a MHRA licence for use here, and therefore cannot be prescribed should they need further supplies. There may be similar medications available here, but excipients may be different, so care and caution is required in prescribing practice. Prescribing as part of a team is imperative here and collaboration with pharmacists, medical and specialist colleagues is required. It may be indicated that a medication review and new regime has been commenced. In the absence of information on excipients in the most up-to-date BNF or in the product literature, contact the manufacturer, as it is essential to ensure that the details are correct (BNF, 2017). Information on product literature can be accessed at www.medicines.org.uk/emc.

Social and Community Networks

Dahlgren and Whitehead's (1991) model considers social and community networks (**Figure 3.3**). This is significant in prescribing practice as these factors will influence a person's ability to participate in their prescribed treatment plan. For example, older people may require a support network in order to be able to participate in shared decision making and undertaking a prescribed medication regime. This support network could be either informal, in the form of family support for decision making, or more formal, in the form third sector initiatives such as community transport to access follow-up appointments or to access medication. This could also include formal networks such as the community pharmacy and medication delivery systems. This is not limited to the elderly; people undergoing therapy for rehabilitation for intravenous drug use often rely on formal community pharmacy initiatives for medication management to support success. Insulin-dependent diabetics and people at the end of their life often need formal community networks such as district nursing services as well as informal family and carer support. Investigating these social and community networks will assist you in person-centred decision making as it will elicit what options a person may have on which to base an informed choice in relation to their care.

General Socio-economic, Cultural and Environmental Conditions

Work, unemployment, food, housing and living conditions have been discussed as part of the social assessment in prescribing practice. Wider strategic considerations identified by Dahlgren and Whitehead (1991) include the following:

Education

Health literacy has a big impact on prescribing practice. A person's knowledge about their condition and the treatment required will assist in the shared prescribing decision-making process. Good health literacy will also impact on a patient's willingness, motivation or ability to undertake a medication regime as prescribed, or whether there could be some deviance from the prescribed regime due to a lack of understanding.

People in education may have reasons for not seeking health professionals on a regular basis if they are transient between addresses, and may let problems lapse. As younger people in education may change addresses from term to holiday time, this can make the follow up of prescribing decisions can also be harder to facilitate. Younger people may not see their health as a priority and may not seek help, especially for potentially embarrassing problems. It is the responsibility of a skilled practitioner to elicit the presenting complaint in a patient-centred consultation in order to identify the problem and plan a collaborative treatment regime.

Water and Sanitation

This is an important consideration in all areas of healthcare practice, as well as in prescribing practice. Consideration of access to clean sanitised areas and clean water supplies is a consideration in prescribing decisions. It is essential to consider if the person has access to adequate facilities with which to self-care effectively, but also to undertake prescribed medication regimes. For example, a patient with psoriasis requiring regular welt bandages and emollient application will need washing facilities in order to be able to undertake this. Sanitation is an important consideration in primary care when making prescribing decisions. It needs to be considered if the person is able to maintain independence in living with an addition medication or treatment regime, and if it is safe to do so. The risk to visiting healthcare and social care professionals in unsanitary living accommodation needs to be considered, as well as the risk to the person. With more and more intravenous therapy being delivered in the home, such as IV antibiotics for cellulitis, it is essential that the risk/benefit ratio is calculated as part of a risk assessment where there is potential harm that could come to the patient if the home were not suitable for visiting healthcare professionals to deliver aseptic care.

Healthcare Services

A lack of access to healthcare services may put pressure on some prescribers when a number of complaints are saved for one short consultation, as with increased demand on health services, the patient may have trouble in accessing appointments. This may also result in patients asking for prescribed medication that is outside of the scope of your prescribing practice. The advanced paramedic practitioner needs to be confident in refusing to prescribe when this occurs in order to ensure patient safety and to protect their registration. For some people, travelling to the health services can be a barrier in terms of timely access for treatment.

Box 3.2 – Must dos for safe prescribing

♦ Right patient? Check your records are the person's records! This sounds simple, but mistakes are easy to make and hard to resolve.
♦ Is the patient's history and presenting complaint appropriate for your scope of prescribing practice? If not, refer on.
♦ Check the patient's weight where appropriate for safe prescribing.
♦ Ascertain allergies or interactions.
♦ Ensure that the patient is not experiencing a condition that may be exacerbated by the medication you wish to prescribe (e.g. NSAIDs with peptic ulcer, antacids, grapefruit and interactions).
♦ Ensure that the patient does not need a modified or reduced dose (e.g. if a child, elderly or in renal failure).
♦ Inform the patient of nuisance and serious side-effects, and what to do and who to see in the event of these occurring.
♦ Pregnancy! This is a high-risk group to prescribe for. Always check for pregnancy in women of a childbearing age.
♦ Be sure you have knowledge of the clinical evidence-based guidelines and local formularies.
♦ Consider de-prescribing and the high-risk danger drugs which have an increased chance of interactions (such as warfarin, NSAIDs, phenytoin, bisphosphonates and antacids).

Similarly, it is essential to consider in your prescribing decision making what healthcare and social care services are available to your patient group, and where you can refer them to for adjuncts to the medication you prescribe. Each local area will commission different services and this can be a challenge for practitioners to keep up-to-date. Offering patients advice on wider holistic and social interventions that they may be able to access, whether commissioned or not in the local area, will ensure that the public health initiative of making every contact count is undertaken within your prescribing role (NHS England, 2014), rather than just the provision of a prescription. **Box 3.2** includes some key points or 'must do's' to guide you in every patient encounter you have in a prescribing context.

Conclusion

In health assessment and consultation for prescribing practice, a key theme that has been discussed in this chapter is the process of a patient-centred and shared decision-making approach to your prescribing practice. While undertaking prescribing practice as a paramedic, there is a high chance that there will be pressure put upon you to undertake prescribing decisions quickly from all stakeholders with whom you will come into contact. As an independent prescriber, it is imperative that you maintain your scope of prescribing practice, prescribing only medicines and drugs that you are competent and confident to prescribe, and for disease processes and pathophysiology that you are familiar with. Prescribing and de-prescribing is a complex business that requires time, caution, attention and practice. Using a consultation framework that is evidence-based, such as the *Competency Framework for All Prescribers* (RPS, 2016), will ensure a structured and cohesive approach to your prescribing practice, where you will be able to demonstrate your ability to meet the competencies in a safe and effective approach.

Key Points of This Chapter

♦ The importance of shared decision-making and a patient-centred approach is central to obtaining a thorough accurate health assessment of your patient.
♦ Various models and frameworks have been explained that may assist you.
♦ It is not always essential to prescribe; it is just as important to consider other options.
♦ Always use and review the 'must do's' for prescribing.

References

Association of Ambulance Chief Executives (2013). *UK Ambulance Services Clinical Practice Guidelines 2013 Pocket Book: Pain Assessment Model.* Bridgwater: Class Professional Publishing.

Blaber, A.Y. and Harris, G. (2016). *Assessment Skills for Paramedics.* Second edition. Maidenhead: Open University Press.

British National Formulary (BNF) (2017). *The British National Formulary 74, September 2017–March 2018.* London: BMJ Group.

College of Paramedics (2018). *Practice Guidance for Paramedic Independent and Supplementary Prescribers.* Bridgwater: College of Paramedics.

Dahlgren, G. and Whitehead, M. (1991). *Policies and Strategies to Promote Social Equity in Health.* Stockholm: Institute of Future Studies.

Elstien, A.S. and Scharz, A. (2002). Clinical problem solving and diagnostic decision making: selective review of the cognitive literature. *British Medical Journal*, 324(7339): 729–32.

Holley-Moore G. and Beach, B. (2016). *Drink Wise, Age Well: Alcohol use and the over 50s in the UK*. London: International Longevity Centre.

Meerabeau, L. and Wright, K. (eds) (2011). *Long-Term Conditions, Nursing Care and Management*. Chichester: Blackwell Publishing.

National Institute for Health and Clinical Excellence (NICE) (2009). *Depression in Adults (Update). Depression: The treatment and management of depression in adults. National Clinical Practice Guideline 90*. London: NICE.

National Prescribing Centre (NPC) (1999). *Nurse Prescribing Bulletin. Signposts for prescribing nurses: General principles of good prescribing*. London: NPC.

Neighbour, R. (1987). *The Inner Consultation: How to develop effective and intuitive consulting style*. Lancaster: MTP Press.

NHS England (2014). *An Implementation Guide and Toolkit for Making Every Contact Count: Using every opportunity to achieve health and well being in the NHS*. London: NHS England.

Nuttall, D. and Rutt-Howland, J. (2011). *The Textbook of Non-Medical Prescribing*, Wiley-Blackwell.

Pendleton, D., Scofield, T. and Tate, P. (1984). *The Consultation: An approach to learning and teaching*. Oxford: Oxford University Press.

Phillips, J. 2007. *Care*. Cambridge: Polity.

Royal Pharmaceutical Society (RPS) (2016). *The Competency Framework for All Prescribers*. London: RPS.

Silverman, J., Kurtz, S. and Draper, J. (1998). *Skills for Communicating with Patients*. Oxford: Radcliffe Medical Press.

Snodden, J. (2009). *Case Management of Long-Term Conditions: Principles and practice for nurses*. Chichester: Blackwell Publishing.

Wingerchuk, D.M. (2012). Smoking: effects on multiple sclerosis susceptibility and disease progression. *Therapeutic Advances in Neurological Disorders*, 5(1): 13–22.

Chapter 4
Basics of Pharmacology

Jennifer Whibley

> ## In This Chapter
>
> - Introduction
> - Key terminology
> - Drug design and delivery
> - Pharmacodynamics
> - Pharmacokinetics
> - Dose response and steady state
> - Conclusion
> - Key points of this chapter
> - References and further reading
> - Useful websites

Introduction

As a prescriber, you need to understand pharmacology; that is, how drugs interact with the body. This includes the mechanisms by which drugs produce a response, as well as how they are processed and eventually removed by the body. At a basic level, we can think of pharmacology as the journey of a medicine through the body. For example, if a tablet is swallowed, how does it actually get to where it needs to go at the concentration needed to produce a therapeutic response? When it gets there, how does the drug produce a response at a cellular level and why is this important? Once it has done its job, how is the drug processed and then removed by the body?

There are formularies and guidelines that have an important role in clinical decision making, but in practice patients are often not straightforward. They may be prescribed multiple medicines for a range of co-morbidities or perhaps have a condition that changes how drugs are processed, as in renal impairment. Understanding how these medicines interact with the body and each other is fundamental in supporting effective clinical decision making in these patients.

The aim of this chapter is to give you a grounding in the basics of the topic. It begins by giving an overview of pharmacology and considering how drugs are

Table 4.1 – Summary of key pharmacology terms

Term	Definition
Affinity	The tendency for a drug to bind to a receptor
Agonist	A drug that **activates** the activity of a receptor producing a change in a physiological system
Antagonist	A drug that **inhibits** the activity of a receptor by blocking the production of a response by an agonist
Bioavailability	The fraction or percentage of drug that reaches the systemic circulation unchanged
Bioequivalence	Drug products that are formulated in a way that they are generally considered therapeutically interchangeable
Dose-response curve	The relationship between the dose of a drug and the pharmacological response
Drug target	The protein (or occasionally DNA, mRNA) that a drug binds to producing a physiological effect. These proteins are often receptors (e.g. ion channels, enzymes or nuclear receptors)
Efficacy	The tendency for a drug to activate the receptor when bound
ED_{50}	The dose that produces 50% of the maximal response of a drug
E_{max}	The dose that produces the maximal response of a drug
Formulation	The process by which a medicinal product is made that can be administered to a patient from the active ingredient and other chemical compounds
Partial agonist	An agonist that produces a maximal response that is less than the maximal response produced by a full agonist
Pharmacodynamics	The field of study concerned with what drugs do to the body
Pharmacokinetics	The field of study concerned with what the body does to drugs
Potency	The concentration of drug needed to produce a defined level of response
Specificity	How selectively a drug will bind to a particular receptor
$T_{1/2}$ (Drug half-live)	The time taken for the concentration of drug to decrease to 50%
Volume of distribution (Vd)	The volume of plasma that would be necessary to account for the total amount of a drug in the patient's body, if that drug were present throughout the body at the same concentration as found in the plasma.

designed and developed. This is followed by sections on the two main branches of the discipline: pharmacodynamics and pharmacokinetics. Examples are given using a range of commonly used drugs to link the concepts covered to clinical practice. The aim is that you will then be able to apply the concepts included in this chapter to any drug within your scope of practice, supporting safe and effective prescribing.

Key Terminology

It is likely that readers of this book will have differing levels of background knowledge of pharmacology, but even if you have some knowledge, the information can act as a refresher.

The summary of key terminology is given in **Table 4.1** to allow you to reflect on your existing knowledge. Are these terms you have heard before? Sometimes terms like 'efficacy' and 'potency' get used, but it is clear that they have not been fully understood. Take a minute to consider your own understanding.

If you feel that you know nothing and the summary in **Table 4.1** makes no sense yet, do not worry – we cover all these terms in this chapter.

Drug Design and Delivery

Before concentrating on the more detailed aspects of pharmacology, it is worth considering a few basic principles of drug design and delivery.

A good place to start this is by defining pharmacology.

Pharmacology is:

'The study of the effects of drugs on the function of living systems.'

(Rang et al, 2016, p. 25)

Humans have known for a long time that compounds can be used to produce an effect on living systems. The Greeks and Romans wrote pharmacopeias listing the uses of many herbal compounds. Until relatively recently, the main way in which treatments were assessed was empirically – observing what effect a treatment had following administration. There was, however, a lack of understanding of how exactly the treatment achieved its therapeutic effect.

Modern pharmacology focuses on understanding how drugs work at a physiological level, meaning that drugs can be targeted specifically and designed to optimise therapeutic outcomes (see **Box 4.2**). The key elements of pharmacology are stated in **Box 4.1**. Importantly, this understanding also helps to minimise toxicity and side-effects.

Box 4.1 – Key elements of pharmacology

♦ The study of drug action.
♦ The study of the chemical constitution of drugs.
♦ The study of their effects on cells and tissues.
♦ The study of their use to treat illness and disease.

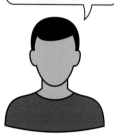

When prescribing for a patient what is it we essentially hope to achieve?

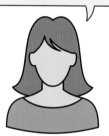

A particular therapeutic response, with the minimum of adverse effects

Box 4.2 – An example of how modern pharmacology can be used to optimise therapeutic outcomes

Opioids act on targets in the body that produce analgesia and have been used for centuries for that purpose. However, they do not act specifically on the targets linked to pain and so produce side-effects, such as constipation and respiratory depression. Modern synthetic opioid-based drugs, such as tramadol and fentanyl, have been developed so that they act more specifically on the receptors linked to analgesia.

This has been achieved through:

♦ knowledge of the chemical structure of the drugs
♦ knowledge of how the drug acts to produce an analgesic response
♦ knowledge of other body systems and how they are affected by the drug.

Is it a Drug or a Medicine?

We tend to use the terms 'drug' and 'medicine' interchangeably, but in this section, we will briefly consider what the differences are between the two. Whilst in practice such semantics may not seem particularly significant, understanding how drugs are 'packaged' into medicines is important in terms of understanding how they ultimately produce a pharmacological affect.

A **drug** is a chemical, other than a nutrient, that produces a biological response in a living organism. This means that poisons are drugs, because a biological response is not necessarily a therapeutic response. As can be seen from overdoses, most drugs that we use therapeutically produce a toxic response when given in sufficient quantities.

A **medicine** is a chemical preparation that contains drugs formulated to produce a therapeutic response at the dose included in the medicine. So, it contains a therapeutic level of drug, but it will almost always contain other ingredients too.

The process of making a drug into a medicine that can be administered to a patient is called 'formulation'. The different types of products including the same drug are called formulations (see **Box 4.3** for an example). Many drugs are available in a variety of formulations that can be selected depending on the patient's needs. Always remember that the 'package' in which the drug comes can mean that it has slightly different pharmacological properties. We will discuss some of the implications of formulation in the pharmacokinetics section on routes of administration.

Box 4.3 – An example of formulations of paracetamol that are available

♦ Tablet
♦ Capsule
♦ Dispersible tablet
♦ IV solution
♦ Oral solution
♦ Suppositories

There are many ingredients that can be used in formulating medicines to help make them suitable for patients to use. A few examples you may see listed in the Summary of Product Characteristics (SPC) are listed in **Table 4.2**.

Table 4.2 – Examples of some of the types of ingredients used in formulation

Ingredient	Purpose
Excipient	Pharmacologically inactive substances, which can be used for a wide range of purposes – for example, as a bulking agent in tablets or coating for modified release preparations
Stabiliser	To physically and chemically stabilise labile drugs so that they do not break down during manufacture and storage
Solvent	A substance that can dissolve a drug so it can be made in to a solution

Pharmacodynamics

The human body is an amazingly complex biological structure with a vast network of mechanisms that control its physiological functions. As we saw in the previous section, drugs are designed to interact with these mechanisms in order to produce a response. However, the complexity of the body means that no drugs work entirely selectively to produce only the intended therapeutic response. This is one of the challenges when developing new drugs as there can be unexpected consequences when drugs begin to be used *in vivo* that have not been encountered during *in vitro* testing. In this section, we will consider how drugs interact with the body to produce a response and will introduce pharmacological principles that are important when prescribing.

Pharmacodynamics: what the drug does to the body

Mechanisms of Drug Action

Drugs are chemicals that interact with drug targets to produce their responses. These targets are often receptors, and so the label of drug–receptor interactions is often used to describe these interactions; see **Box 4.4**.

Box 4.4 – Examples of physiological responses that can be produced through drug–receptor interactions

♦ Change in contractility of a tissue, e.g. muscle.
♦ Change in excitability of neurons and thus neural stimulation.
♦ Changes in gene transcription.

The extent of change caused by the drug depends on both its **affinity** and **efficacy**.

Drug–Receptor Interactions

As the schematic **Figure 4.1** shows, the shape of the drug and the target are what defines whether the drug binds to the receptor and produces a response. In drug development there is a significant amount of work which goes into designing and then refining the chemical structure to optimise the shape to get the best possible fit.

These interactions are often described using the lock and key hypothesis, and we can imagine this like the shape of a key used to open a lock. The key is made up of a whole range of cuts and groves, giving it a unique 3D shape. Other keys might fit partially into the lock, but it is only the one shape that will open it fully.

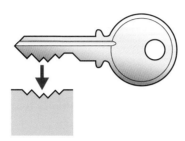

Figure 4.1 – Diagram showing the 'lock and key' hypothesis

Drugs are designed to take advantage of this principle, either by binding to activate the receptor or instead occupying the receptor binding site to prevent binding of endogenous chemicals:

♦ Drugs that are designed to fit the lock and activate a physiological process are known as **agonists**.
♦ Drugs that are designed to block the lock from binding chemicals that can activate them are known as **antagonists** (see **Figure 4.2**).

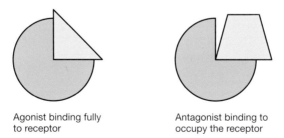

Agonist binding fully
to receptor

Antagonist binding to
occupy the receptor

Figure 4.2 – Diagram showing differences between agonist and antagonist binding

For example, antihistamines are antagonists that attach to histamine receptors, blocking endogenous histamine from causing an allergic reaction.

Affinity, Efficacy, Specificity and Potency

These terms are often used interchangeably yet they represent very different pharmacological concepts. Before looking at the other types of drug interactions it is worth focusing in more detail on these terms to make sure they are clear.

Affinity is the tendency for a drug to bind to a receptor. It can be thought of in basic terms of how attracted the molecule is to the receptor binding site. Thinking of an example, we may have two drugs both of which produce an equal response when bound to a receptor but one is much more strongly attracted than the other to this receptor. The one that is more strongly attracted is said to have a higher affinity for the drug target and it is likely this one will produce a greater effect in vivo because it will bind much more readily with the target.

Efficacy is the tendency of the drug to produce a response when bound to a receptor. As we have seen the shape of the drug and the receptor play a key role in this. A drug may have a high affinity for a receptor but have no efficacy, so it really wants to bind with the receptor but produces no response when it does. These in fact are generally the key characteristics of an antagonist – high affinity but no efficacy. Conversely what we are usually aiming for with an agonist is a high affinity and a high efficacy.

Specificity is how selectively a drug binds to a particular receptor. It is important to realise that in the body there a whole host of structurally similar receptors that regulate quite different physiological responses. Often drugs will bind to more than one receptor subtype. Ideally a drug will have a high level of specificity as this will reduce the likelihood of side effects. Interestingly, however, the lack of specificity of some drugs has led to them being used for other indications than those they were originally licensed for.

Potency refers to the amount of drug required to produce a defined level of response. If for example 1mg of Drug A produces the same response as 10mg of Drug B, then we can see that Drug A is more potent. This does not mean it is 'stronger' per se but merely that you need less drug to produce a particular therapeutic response.

Other Types of Drug Interactions

Whilst agonists and antagonists are the most common types of drug interactions, it is important to be aware that there are several others.

Partial Agonists

As the name suggests, these drugs bind to receptors, leading to partial activation of a physiological response. This may be useful when it is necessary to produce a smaller response than a full agonist would.

For example, buprenorphine is a partial agonist of μ-opioid receptors and one of its uses is supporting opioid-dependent patients when withdrawing from opioids. When administered, it produces a response, but as the graph in **Figure 4.3** shows, not of the same magnitude as opioids such as heroin that are full agonists of μ-opioid receptors.

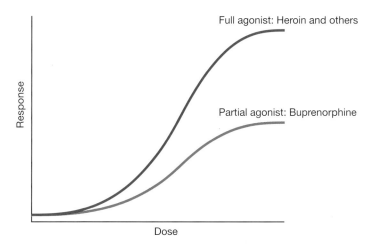

Figure 4.3 – Graph showing effect of buprenorphine as a partial agonist versus heroin

As a partial agonist, the maximum effect of an equivalent dose of buprenorphine is less than that of a full agonist such as morphine or heroin.

Competitive and Non-competitive Antagonists

Competitive antagonists compete with other agents to occupy receptor binding sites. The two-way arrow in **Figure 4.4** highlights that this is a reversible effect and depends on the affinity that both the agonist and antagonist have for the receptor binding site. Some drugs, such as naloxone can displace other molecules from the receptor binding site, as illustrated in **Figure 4.4**. Other competitive antagonists merely compete with other molecules to occupy the binding site.

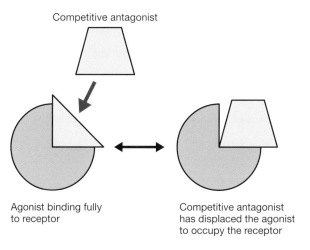

Figure 4.4 – Diagram showing action of competitive antagonists

Naloxone is a competitive agonist that acts to displace both agonists and partial agonists at opioid receptors. It has essentially no pharmacological activity in the absence of opioids and is used to treat an opioid overdose.

Non-competitive antagonists are different in that they bind irreversibly to the receptor binding site, as illustrated in **Figure 4.5**. This means that the only way for the effect of the antagonist to be overcome is when the receptor itself is broken down and replaced.

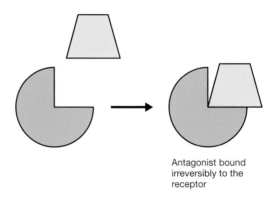

Antagonist bound
irreversibly to the
receptor

Figure 4.5 – Diagram showing action of non-competitive antagonists

For example, aspirin is a non-competitive antagonist. Its use as an antiplatelet for chronic prophylaxis is due to irreversible binding to receptors on platelets. Platelets have a lifespan of ten days, which could potentially lead to problems with the effect lasting the lifetime of the platelet. However, the risk is minimised as only low doses are used for this indication and because platelets are replenished from the bone marrow daily.

Inverse Agonists

Drugs known as inverse agonists produce a net decrease in the basal activity of the receptor with which they interact. To understand this concept, we must first understand the concept of a two-state model of receptors. This model suggests that receptors exist in two different conformational states, effectively meaning they exist in two different 3D shapes. One shape is a resting state where the receptor is essentially inactive. The shape, however, changes when the receptor is active and able to produce a response, as **Figure 4.6** shows. Normally they exist in an equilibrium between the two states.

An inverse agonist has a greater affinity for the resting state of the receptor and so binds more readily to the receptor in this state. Once the inverse agonist is bound to the receptor, it is unable to change into the active conformation, causing the equilibrium between active and inactive to shift in favour of the inactive. The net effect is to reduce the number of active receptors, thus causing an overall decrease in the basal physiological activity.

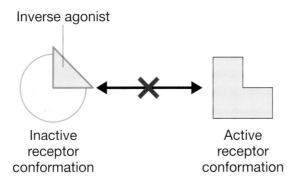

Figure 4.6 – Diagram showing action of inverse agonist, two-state model

Allosteric Interactions

Allosteric sites are secondary binding sites on receptors that can change the affinity of molecules for the primary binding site, as can be seen in **Figure 4.7**. They do this by causing the shape of the binding site to change. This can mean that other molecules may either be more or less likely to bind and cause a response.

An example of this is the drug cinnacalet (brand name Mimpara). This drug is licensed for treatment of hyperparathyroidism and works by binding to an allosteric site on the calcium sensing receptor on the surface of the chief cell of the parathyroid gland.

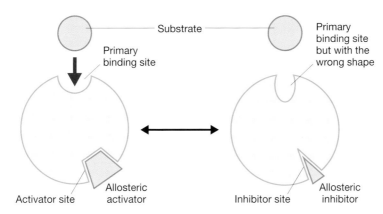

Figure 4.7 – Diagram showing allosteric interactions

This causes the receptor to have increased sensitivity to extracellular calcium, which consequently leads to a reduction in circulating parathyroid hormone.

For more information, see the SPC at https://www.medicines.org.uk/emc/product/5599#.

Types of Drug Targets

Ligand Gated Ion Channels

These transmembrane channels regulate the passage of ions, such as Na^+, K^+ and Cl^-, into and out of cells. They open and close in response to the binding of a chemical messenger or ligand. These ligands can be drugs, which either activate or inhibit opening of the channels by binding directly to the channel or an intermediary receptor. Drugs that act on these receptors tend to be fast acting because the channels they interact with are those that neurotransmitters work on (see **Figure 4.8**).

For example:

♦ **Local anaesthetics**: block sodium (Na^+) channels thus stopping conduction of pain signals.
♦ **Nifedipine**: blocks receptors on calcium channels in arterioles, hence it is in the class of drugs that are known as calcium channel blockers.
♦ **Drugs that act on GABA modulated Cl⁻ channels**: GABA is the predominant inhibitory neurotransmitter in the brain. GABA receptors regulate the influx of Cl⁻ in to cells, leading to stabilisation of tissue because depolarisation is difficult in the presence of these negatively charged ions. There are several drugs which utilise this system by interacting with GABA receptors, e.g. benzodiazepines and other antiepileptic drugs.

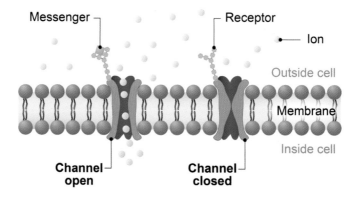

Figure 4.8 – Showing action of a ligand-gated ion channel

Source: © designua / 123RF

G-Protein-Coupled Receptors (GPCRs)

These receptors are coupled with proteins known as a G-proteins, which consist of seven transmembrane segments (see **Figure 4.9**) linked to intracellular G-proteins. They conduct signals through their coupling with intracellular systems. Extracellular binding therefore activates a cascade that leads to a change in intracellular processes. These receptors are widely spread through the body and act to regulate a whole host of physiological responses. Drugs acting on these receptors also produce a relatively rapid response, but because of the time taken to transduce the signal, the response is slower than is the case for drugs acting on ion channels.

For example, opioids act on G-protein-coupled receptors that are linked to various signalling pathways and modulation of physiological processes.

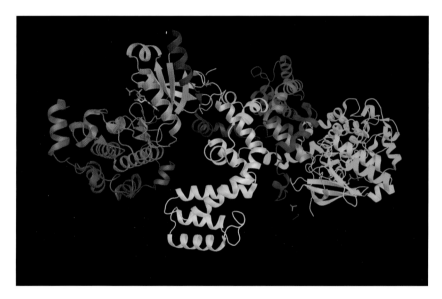

Figure 4.9 – Diagram showing action of GPCRs and a 3D image of the structure of a GPCR, Kinase 6

Source: © Iculig / 123RF.

Enzyme-Coupled Receptors

These act in a similar way to GPCRs, in that an enzyme is involved in conducting the signal intracellularly. However, the way in which the signal is conducted by the enzyme is different (see **Figure 4.10**). In its inactive state the enzyme consists of two separate molecules. Binding of a ligand, such as a drug or a hormone, to an extracellular binding site causes the separate intracellular kinase domain to associate. This leads to phosphorylation of the intracellular kinase, which allows these to act as docking sites for other intracellular proteins. This ultimately leads to a cellular response.

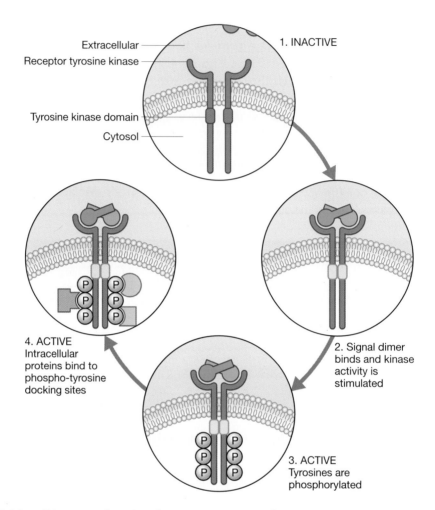

Figure 4.10 – Diagram showing how enzyme-couple receptors work using the example of tyrosine kinase receptors

Insulin is an example of a drug that exerts its effects through this type of receptor. Because of the fact that it acts through a cascade of secondary molecules these type of interactions can take up to several hours to produce a response.

Nuclear or Intracellular Receptors

These receptors are found within the cell and exist unbound either in the cytoplasm or the nucleus. Those that exist in the cytoplasm move within the nucleus after binding with a ligand as they require access to DNA to produce their response. When activated, they cause changes in gene expression and therefore protein synthesis (see **Figure 4.11**). Because of this, it can take hours or days to see a response.

Examples of nuclear or intracellular receptors include hormones such as testosterone and oestrogen, as well as glucocorticoid steroids.

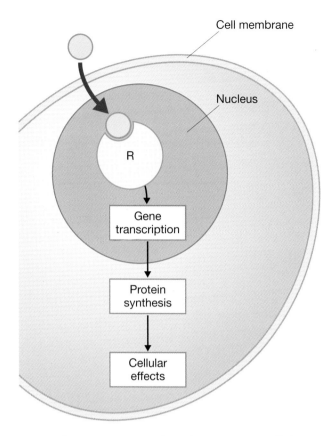

Figure 4.11 – Diagram showing action of nuclear or intracellular receptors

Self-test exercise

- What is the difference between affinity and efficacy?
- What pharmacological and biological properties lead to drugs causing side-effects?
- How do dose and response differ between full, partial and inverse agonists, as well as antagonists?
- What are the main types of drug targets?

Finally, think about some of the drugs you will be prescribing and spend some time looking at their pharmacodynamic properties. You can find this information at: https://www.medicines.org.uk/emc. Use the search function to look up drugs relevant to your practice. When you click on the monograph for a drug you will see it is split into different sections, one of which is the pharmacodynamic properties of that medicine.

Pharmacokinetics

Pharmacokinetics helps describe the journey of the drug into, around and then out of the body. It is hugely important to understand the pharmacokinetic factors that influence this journey as they affect patients in a whole host of ways in practice, for example, in choosing the right formulation, doing appropriate monitoring and switching between medicines.

> **Pharmacokinetics:** what the body does to the drug

There are the four key areas of pharmacokinetics that are used to characterise what happens to the drug *in vivo*. The mnemonic ADME can help you to remember these four key areas (see **Box 4.5**).

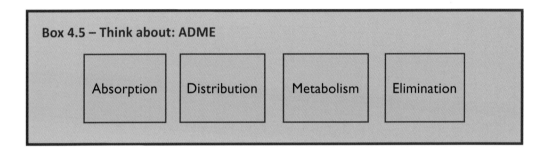

Box 4.5 – Think about: ADME

| Absorption | Distribution | Metabolism | Elimination |

Absorption

Drugs must cross lipid bilayers to reach their site of action. This process of a drug moving from site of administration into the systemic circulation is known as absorption. The complexity of this process depends on the route of administration. For example, absorption of drugs given orally depends on the drug not being degraded in the gastrointestinal (GI) tract, as well as the ability to cross the intestinal epithelium. Drugs given intravenously bypass these problems. In this section we will look at the physiological and physicochemical factors that are important in absorption.

General Considerations

The rate and extent of absorption depends on a number of factors and is influenced by how medicines are formulated and the route of administration chosen (see **Box 4.6** for details).

> **Box 4.6 – Some factors affecting the rate and extent of absorption**
>
> **Physiological factors:**
>
> ♦ Blood flow to the site of absorption
> ♦ The total surface area available for absorption
> ♦ Contact time at the absorption site
>
> **Physicochemical factors:**
>
> ♦ Drug solubility
> ♦ Drug chemical stability
> ♦ Lipid-to-water partition coefficient
> ♦ Degree of ionisation of the drug

Routes of Administration

There are a whole range of routes by which drugs can be administered. The main ones are:

♦ Oral
♦ Intravenous
♦ Subcutaneous/intramuscular
♦ Topical – including application to epithelial surfaces (such as the skin, nasal mucosa, cornea and vagina)
♦ Transdermal – this is topical form of administration where drugs are applied to the skin using patches for sustained release of drugs in to the systemic circulation
♦ Sublingual
♦ Rectal
♦ Inhalation

For each of these, there are a range of factors that influence the rate and extent of absorption of different drugs.

Table 4.3 gives an overview of some of the factors affecting the absorption of drugs via different routes of administration.

Table 4.3 – Some factors affecting the absorption of drugs

Route	Physiological factor	Physicochemical factor	Examples
Oral	Gastric emptying rate Gastric motility Changes in gastric pH as this affects drug ionisation Whether there is an active transport process for the drug	Particle size Formulation, e.g. tablet requires dissolution, liquid does not Lipid solubility Degree of ionisation	This is the most common route of administration and most products are available orally Note the variety of formulations available that manipulate physiological factors e.g. modified release and enteric coated medicines
Intravenous	This bypasses the need for absorption across a membrane, so IV drugs have 100% bioavailability	Particle size Excipients must not cause irritation at injection site	Vancomycin – when given orally, it is not absorbed in the GI tract and only has a local action
Subcutaneous/ intramuscular	Local perfusion of tissues and the site of injection affect absorption Increased perfusion can cause more rapid absorption (e.g. following exercise) Decreased perfusion can slow absorption (e.g. heart failure)	Formulation can be used to delay release of drugs, e.g. depot injections of drugs for mental health and contraception	Paliperidone IM injection lasts three months due to low water solubility leading to slow release
Topical	Often used for local action Systemic absorption may occur and must be considered when prescribing	Barrier that epithelial and cutaneous tissue presents to absorption Drugs must have low molecular weight and high lipid solubility for this route	Steroid creams used in treating local inflammation Eye drops and nasal sprays are considered topical as applied to epithelial tissue

Route	Physiological factor	Physicochemical factor	Examples
Transdermal	A form of topical administration where patches are formulated for sustained release of drug in to the systemic crculation Skin is a significant barrier for drugs to cross Useful where consistent serum levels of the drug are required	Only suitable for lipid soluble because of the lipid nature of the skin	Opioid derivatives, e.g. fentanyl and buprenorphine; hormone patches
Sublingual	Allows fast absorption across the mucosal membrane of the mouth	Useful when drugs are extensively metabolised by liver enzymes/ unstable at gastric pH	Glyceryl trinitrate; Lorazepam tablets used off licence in acute anxiety to avoid parenteral administration
Rectal	Useful in patients where oral access is a problem, e.g. vomiting or Nil by Mouth Good absorption via this route and can minimise the effects of first pass metabolism (see explanation below)	Can be used to achieve a local effect or a systemic effect. The formulation is influenced mainly by this	Suppositories, enemas and foams all available
Inhalation	Useful due to the large absorptive surface area in lungs Local administration for respiratory disease allows smaller doses to be used than via oral administration	Mainly used for administration of locally acting drugs Some volatile gases (e.g. Anaesthetics) are administered by this route	Steroid inhalers; beta-agonist inhalers; gaseous anaesthetics

First Pass Metabolism

Drugs can be metabolised before they even enter the circulation when blood from the small intestine travels via the hepatic portal vein to the liver, before then entering the systemic circulation.

This is known as first pass metabolism and with some drugs the dose is metabolised significantly before it can reach the site of action. This means that there can be a large variation in the serum concentration resulting from a dose given parenterally versus when given orally.

Box 4.7 – Drugs that undergo extensive first pass metabolism

- ♦ Aspirin
- ♦ Glyceryl trinitrate
- ♦ Levodopa
- ♦ Morphine
- ♦ Metoprolol
- ♦ Salbutamol
- ♦ Verapamil

Bioavailability and Area Under the Concentration Time Curve (AUC)

There are several factors that can affect the amount of drug that is absorbed into the systemic circulation. These include the first pass metabolism described above along with others, such as, degradation in gastric acid or the barrier presented by the intestinal mucosa. Often therefore the full dose of a drug given orally does not reach the systemic circulation. This is in contrast with drugs given IV as they are introduced directly in to the systemic circulation.

Bioavailability describes the fraction or percentage of drug that reaches the systemic circulation following oral administration. According to the SPC amoxicillin capsules are approximately 70% bioavailable. This means that only 70% of the oral dose will reach the systemic circulation. The bioavailability of the IV injection will in contrast be 100%.

The AUC looks at the extent of absorption and elimination by sampling serum concentration over time in test subjects. The concentration points are then plotted on a graph against time which gives a curve as concentration rises following administration and then falls as elimination occurs. The resulting area underneath this graphical curve essentially shows the extent to which the drug has been present in the body. These curves are plotted separately following oral and IV administration and the resulting figures are used to estimate bioavailability by dividing AUC oral by AUC intravenous.

Remember!

When switching between routes, there can be differences in absorption, which can be clinically significant, leading to a difference in bioavailability. This is the amount of a drug that reaches the systemic circulation unchanged.

There can also be variations in bioavailability when the same route is used but a different type of formulation, like a tablet or a liquid, is given. For example, **Table 4.4** shows the different dose equivalents between **citalopram** tablets and oral solution.

Table 4.4 – Citalopram doses for different oral formulations

Tablet dose equivalent	Solution
10 mg	8 mg (4 drops)
20 mg	16 mg (8 drops)
30 mg	24 mg (12 drops)
30 mg	32 mg (16 drops)

Some drugs are in fact so prone to variations in bioavailability that even different makes of the same formulation, such as, tablets can show variation in bioavailability that can have a clinical impact. Patients stabilised on these medicines should therefore be prescribed their medication by brand. This is the case with several antiepileptic drugs, for example, guidance from the MHRA suggests that carbamazepine tablets must always be prescribed by brand/branded generic for epilepsy because of differences in bioavailability between formulations.

If, however, there is no clinical impact on substituting one formulation for another, then the formulations can be said to be **bioequivalent**.

Think about...

Is there a clinical difference between the different formulations of drug you will be prescribing?

Self-test exercise

♦ Can you name a drug that you know you must prescribe by brand?
♦ What factors can you think of that might affect the bioavailability of a medicine?
♦ Is there any monitoring you would need to do when switching between formulations?
♦ How would you explain to a patient why the dose of their medication has changed if you switch formulation and there is a dose adjustment (as in the case of citalopram liquid and tablets)?

Distribution

Once the drug has been absorbed, it is distributed around the body. It is important to realise that this distribution will not be uniform due to the complex makeup of the body. In order to describe the distribution of drugs, we must imagine the body as made up of multiple compartments. The different composition of the compartments means that some drugs will naturally partition into some compartments rather than others, leading to variable drug concentrations in different compartments.

Distribution into Body Compartments

The body can be seen as consisting of five main compartments:

♦ intracellular fluid
♦ interstitial fluid
♦ blood plasma
♦ other bodily fluids (e.g. cerebrospinal, intraocular and synovial fluid)
♦ fat.

Factors Affecting Distribution

Drugs can move between the compartments with several factors influencing the rate and extent of this movement. Most distribution occurs through passive diffusion:

♦ **Blood flow to the compartment:** drugs tend to distribute most quickly in areas that are highly perfused. This includes the brain, the lungs and the heart. Over time, lipid soluble drugs will redistribute to areas of fat that are normally poorly perfused.
♦ **Permeability of barriers:** the nature of the barrier separating the compartments is an important factor in terms of how the drugs move between these compartments. One important example of a barrier is the blood-brain barrier (see **Box 4.8**).
♦ **Binding within the compartment:** drugs may become bound to proteins in a compartment, meaning that they are retained within that compartment. There is often extensive binding of the drug to plasma proteins, sometimes with less than 1% of the drug existing unbound and able to produce a pharmacological response.

Changes in the levels of plasma protein and displacement of one drug by another can lead to changes in the levels of the unbound drug (see **Box 4.9**).

♦ **Fat: water partition:** drugs with a high lipid solubility, like morphine, are more likely to cross the blood–brain barrier. Other drugs, like gentamicin, have a low lipid solubility and therefore tend to stay in aqueous compartments. Most drugs have a relatively low fat: water partition and do not extensively partition into fat.

Box 4.8 – Key information about the blood–brain barrier

The blood–brain barrier

♦ The function of the barrier is to protect the brain from damage by circulating chemicals.
♦ Consists of endothelial cells with tight junctions surrounded by pericytes.
♦ Normally impermeable to many drugs and presents a challenge when formulating a medicine whose site of action is within the central nervous system (CNS).
♦ Small, lipid soluble and unionised molecules pass through most readily.
♦ Inflammation can cause the barrier to become 'leaky' as its integrity is compromised. Drugs that would normally not have access can cross. Patients may be at risk of increased side-effects.

Practice example:

♦ Methylnaltrexone is a μ-opioid receptor antagonist used for patients with opioid-induced constipation. It cannot cross the blood–brain barrier due to its low lipid solubility and polarity, and so only antagonises peripheral receptors located in the GI tract responsible for constipation. It cannot act on μ-opioid receptors in the brain so does not interfere with the analgesic effect of opioid.

Box 4.9 – Plasma protein binding

Plasma protein binding

♦ Drugs can bind to binding sites on proteins that exist in the plasma.
♦ If the drug is bound to plasma proteins, then it is not free to interact with the drug target.
♦ Some drugs are extensively bound to proteins and so a large proportion of the dose taken may not reach the target.
♦ Usually this is not a problem as any dose taken takes into account the normal level of protein binding.
♦ However, any reduction in the amount of plasma proteins in the body can lead to a higher than normal serum concentration of the drug.
♦ Clinically significant interactions due to displacement of the bound drug is most likely in drugs with a narrow therapeutic index (see below for more on the therapeutic index).
♦ Albumin is the most important plasma protein involved in binding drugs.

Volume of Distribution (Vd)

Vd can be confusing to understand initially as it refers to a theoretical volume rather than an actual volume per se. It is a concept used to describe the way in which drugs partition in the body by essentially comparing the way in which a drug actually distributes against its concentration in the plasma.

> **Definition:**
>
> The Vd is the volume of plasma that would be necessary to account for the total amount of a drug in the patient's body, if that drug were present throughout the body at the same concentration as found in the plasma.

To illustrate this idea, we can compare two hypothetical drugs (see **Case Study 4.1**).

Case Study 4.1

The examples below are designed to illustrate what information can be gained from determining the Vd in terms of how drugs distribute in the body.

Drug A

500 mcg of Drug A is given to a patient who weighs 70 kg. This drug is relatively water soluble and stays in the plasma. Levels show that peak plasma concentration is 30 mcg/L. In this patient, dividing the initial dose by the plasma concentration shows us that theoretically we would need 16.7 L to distribute the drug throughout the body at the same concentration. If we divide this by 70 kg, then we get a Vd of 0.24 L/kg.

Drug B

500 mcg of Drug B is given to the same patient. This drug is relatively lipid soluble and distributes extensively outside the plasma. Levels show that peak plasma concentration is 1 mcg/L. Dividing the initial dose by plasma concentration shows that we would need 500 L of plasma to distribute the drug throughout the body at the same concentration. Dividing this by 70 kg, we get a Vd of 7.14 L/kg.

We can see that the amount of plasma needed to distribute Drug B is significantly greater than Drug A and so the Vd is much bigger. Whilst a large Vd does not tell us exactly where the drug distributes to, we know that it partitions into tissues or fluids outside of the plasma.

Metabolism

Following absorption and distribution, the concentration of the free drug will begin to decline due to metabolism and elimination:

♦ **Metabolism** is the changing of the chemical structure of the drug by the body to make it easier to excrete. The products of metabolism are metabolites.
♦ **Elimination** is the physical removal of the drug from the body, mainly via urine or faeces.

In this section we will focus on the two types of metabolic reaction, which often happen sequentially, and are called phase 1 and phase 2 reactions.

Phase 1 Reactions

These involve the chemical structure of the drug being altered through chemical reactions – oxidation, reduction or hydrolysis. The resulting metabolites fall into three pharmacological categories:

1. The metabolite has no pharmacological activity of its own.
2. The metabolite retains some pharmacological activity.
3. The metabolite is more pharmacologically active than the drug itself, for example, a prodrug.

The metabolites produced from drugs can therefore have an important role in their own right in the therapeutic action of a medicine.

Prodrugs

These are drugs that require metabolism to become pharmacologically active. It is therefore not the drug but the **metabolite** that acts on a receptor target to produce or inhibit a physiological response. This method of drug delivery is useful for a range of reasons, including helping target drugs to a specific site of action or minimising side-effects.

Box 4.10 – Examples of prodrugs

♦ Codeine is a prodrug of morphine. The codeine is metabolised *in vivo* to morphine.
♦ Enalapril is activated by a phase 1 reaction to enalaprilat.
♦ Azathioprine is metabolised to the active metabolite mercaptopurine.

Think about...

Any drugs you will be prescribing that are either prodrugs or have active metabolites.

What impact could a change in the metabolic capacity of the body have on their therapeutic effects?

Phase 2 Reactions

In phase 2 reactions, the drug or phase 1 metabolite has a molecule attached to it that usually increases its water solubility, making it easier to excrete from the body. The name given to this attachment is conjugation. Unlike phase 1 metabolites, the products of phase 2 reactions do not usually display any pharmacological activity.

The CYP450 Enzyme System

Enzymes play an important role in catalysing drug metabolism. A particularly important group of hepatic enzymes are the CYP450 enzymes. Within this group, there are various subsets of enzymes, known as isoforms, that are responsible for metabolising different drugs.

For example, Carbamazepine is metabolised mainly by the CYP450 isoform CYP450 3A4 into its primary metabolite carbamazepine-10, 11-epoxide.

Changes in the capacity of these enzyme systems can lead to clinically significant changes in drug concentrations. Drugs can act to increase or decrease the amount of CYP450 enzymes, leading to potential drug interactions (see **Table 4.5** for details).

Table 4.5 – Potential drug interactions with CYP450 enzymes

The change is known as...	And the result is...	Example
Enzyme **induction**	**Increased** synthesis of enzymes by the liver	*Carbamazepine, phenytoin, sulphonylureas, rifampicin*
Enzyme **inhibition**	**Decreased** synthesis of enzymes by the liver	*Sodium valproate, cimetidine, ciprofloxacin, metronidazole*

Think about...

♦ Prescribing of drugs that induce or inhibit CYP450 enzymes.
♦ These can lead to significant drug interactions.
♦ Because induction/inhibition can take some time to occur, make sure this is considered, even if a patient presents sometime after the initiation of therapy.

Make you sure you become familiar with any enzyme inducers/inhibitors within your scope of practice

Elimination

Elimination involves the physical removal of a drug or its metabolites from the body. It can happen via the following routes, depending on the lipid/water solubility of the drug.

Routes of excretion:
♦ urine
♦ faeces
♦ sweat
♦ expired air.

Excretion of water-soluble products:
♦ Drugs that undergo hepatic metabolism often produce water-soluble metabolites of lipid soluble drugs.
♦ The water solubility of these metabolites allows them to be renally excreted in the urine. This is the route of excretion of most drugs.
♦ The drug/metabolite may also be excreted in secretions such as sweat or breast milk. In most cases the amount excreted via these routes is small compared to the amount that is excreted renally. It is important to consider breast milk due to the effect that the drug contained in the milk can have on the baby. This is covered in more detail in **Chapter 9**.
♦ The lungs are a site of excretion for some volatile or gaseous drugs, such as anaesthetics

Excretion of lipid-soluble products:
♦ Anything that is not freely water-soluble goes via the bile duct into the gut and is then excreted from the body via the faeces.
♦ A complication of this route is the enterohepatic shunt (also known as enterohepatic circulation), whereby the drug/metabolite excreted in the bile can be reabsorbed from the GI tract, which can prolong its duration of action.

Enterohepatic shunt or circulation

Drugs that have been hepatically metabolised can enter the GI tract in the bile, where the metabolic process can be reversed making the drug active again. For example, drugs that have been conjugated with glucuronides in the liver, can be hydrolysed in the GI tract allowing the drug to re-enter the systemic circulation. This leads to a proportion of recirculating drug prolonging the action of the drug (this can be up to 20% of total drug in the body). Drugs that undergo enterohepatic circulation include morphine and the oestrogen used in contraception, ethinylestradiol.

The Kinetics of Elimination

Drugs can be eliminated at different rates and understanding this can support clinical decision making on, for example, dosing regimens or wash-out periods between drugs.

First Order Kinetics

This is the most straightforward model to understand and is the one that most drugs follow. In this model the rate of metabolism is predictable and proportional to the concentration of the drug present.

Definition:

It can be defined using the plasma half-life ($T_{1/2}$) where:

$T_{1/2}$ = the time taken for the concentration of drug to decrease by 50%

To illustrate this, we can take a hypothetical drug – Drug A:

Imagine a patient has been taking Drug A which has a $T_{1/2}$ of 10 hours. This means it will take ten hours for the concentration of this drug to be reduced by 50% from its peak values. We will therefore see the following pattern of decreasing concentration;

♦ Amount of drug present at time zero = 100%
♦ Amount of drug present at ten hours (one half-life) = 50%
♦ Amount of drug present at twenty hours (two half-lives) = 25%
♦ Amount of drug present at thirty hours (three half-lives) = 12.5%
♦ Amount of drug present at forty hours (four half-lives) = 6.25%
♦ Amount of drug present at fifty hours (five half-lives) = 3.125%

The amount remaining in the body will continue to decrease by 50% every ten hours until there is no drug left in the body. Usually it is considered that it will take approximately five half-lives for a drug to be reduced sufficiently for it to be removed from the body in terms of having any clinical relevance. This makes sense when we consider the information above that shows almost 97% of drug has been removed after five half-lives.

Example: the $T_{1/2}$ of amiodarone is approximately 50 days, although this varies considerably between patients. A $T_{1/2}$ of 100 days has been reported. This means that five half-lives can be anywhere between 250 to 500 days. This information is important as it explains why there is therefore a risk that interactions with other drugs can occur long after treatment has ceased.

Zero Order Kinetics

Some drugs follow unpredictable metabolic kinetics, also known as saturation kinetics. This is because they involve metabolism by enzyme systems that can become saturated.

Imagine a system where there are a finite number of enzymes. On initial administration, the drug will start filling up the enzyme binding sites. However, when all the enzymes are occupied and the system is saturated, then the rate of metabolism is limited. At this point, a small increase in dose can lead to a large increase in drug concentrations. As patients can have varying amounts of metabolic enzymes this can make the point of saturation difficult to predict.

For example, phenytoin undergoes zero order elimination, meaning that a small increase in dose can lead to a significant increase in serum concentration as metabolic enzymes become saturated.

Dose Response and Steady State

In this final section we will look at the relationship between the administration of a dose and the response that is produced.

Dose Response

Figure 4.12 features a graph showing examples of what are known as a dose response curves. These curves represent the typical relationship between the dose administered and the response that is produced. This shows response as a percentage of the maximum response against increasing dose. By plotting these graphs, we can compare the E_{max} and the ED_{50} of different drugs that produce similar effects. **Figure 4.12** also demonstrates how we can use this to plot how types of drugs can affect response – in this instance, how a competitive antagonist affects the dose response of an agonist.

Reminder of what Emax and ED50 represent:

E_{max} : the dose that produces the maximal response of a drug

ED_{50}: the dose that produces 50% of the maximal response of a drug

---

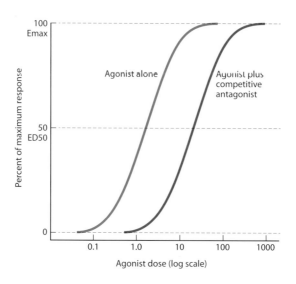

Figure 4.12 – Dose response curve

The response seen with an agonist makes sense when we think of it in the context of a biological system where response relies on drug–receptor interactions. Essentially what the curves show is that at very low doses there is a smaller effect on response. This is because the receptor binding sites are not occupied and only when a sufficient portion of them have been filled is a response seen. Once a sufficient number of binding sites are occupied, then the relationship between dose and response becomes essentially linear, as seen in the middle portion of the curve. At higher doses, the increase in response slows again as binding sites become increasingly filled and it is harder at this point for the agonist to find a vacant receptor site to bind.

When a competitive antagonist is added to the system, we see a shift in the agonist dose response curve to the right. The maximal response that can be produced (E_{max}) does not change, but a higher dose is required to produce that response. The reason for this is that the effect of competitive antagonists can be overcome.

Example: to understand the relevance of this in practice, it may help to think about what impact this can have in the body.

Imagine there is an agonist that is actually an endogenous product – let's say a hormone – and there is a certain amount circulating in the body. If we imagine that the amount in circulation leads to a response that is equivalent to the ED_{50}, then under normal circumstances 50% of the maximal response will be produced. If we then administer a drug that is a competitive antagonist of this hormone, then it will mean that the circulating dose of hormone will no longer be able to produce 50% of the maximal response. However, if the body then increased production of this hormone to compensate, it would compete with the antagonist and the response could again reach the ED_{50}.

The addition of a competitive antagonist is only one example of how dose response can change, which should make sense when we think of the different types of drug receptor interactions there can be.

Antagonist alone: antagonists have no efficacy as they block the actions of agonists. If you plot a dose response curve of the antagonist alone, it will therefore be flat as no matter how much you increase the dose, no response will be seen (refer back to **Figure 4.3** for an illustration of this).

Partial agonists: these drugs produce a maximal response that is less than the maximal response produced by a full agonist. This means that the E_{max} and ED_{50} will both be less (refer back to **Figure 4.3** for an illustration of this).

Inverse agonist: as these produce a negative effect, the dose response curve becomes inverted into negative values.

A full discussion of all the ways in which dose response can be altered by various agonists/antagonists is beyond the scope of this book; for further reading, please see one of the pharmacology textbooks listed in the references and further reading section.

Steady State

It is important to remember that *in vivo* the drug is interacting with a whole range of processes and is normally given as repeated doses. This leads to a balance between the amount being administered and the amount being excreted. **Figure 4.13** shows a graph that illustrates what happens with repeated administration.

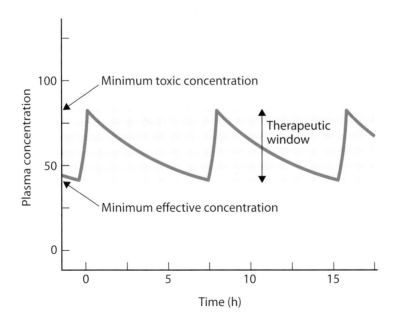

Figure 4.13 – Graph showing repeated administration

What this shows is that with repeated dosing, there are fluctuations in plasma concentration over time; these are known as the peak and trough plasma concentrations. These are linked to factors such as how rapidly the dose is absorbed and distributed, metabolised and excreted. Despite these inevitable fluctuations, the peaks and troughs are consistent, meaning that on average the plasma concentration is at a level known as steady state.

Steady state is reached when the rate of absorption equals the rate of elimination.

It is important to appreciate that when a drug is initiated serum levels do not immediately reach steady state. Thinking back to how drugs work, this is not surprising. Because metabolism and elimination occur following administration, several doses are usually needed to build up the concentrations at the receptor sites to produce the therapeutic levels needed.

Steady state is therefore usually reached after approximately three to five half-lives.

For example;

♦ Drug A has a half-life of 5 hours, so steady state will be reached after approximately 15–25 hours.
♦ Drug B has a half-life of 20 hours, so steady state will be reached after approximately 60–100 hours.

As well as steady state, **Figure 4.13** also highlights another pharmacological key term: therapeutic window (or therapeutic index). This term defines the range of serum concentrations at which a therapeutic response is seen. It is discussed further in the next section on therapeutic drug monitoring.

Key Points

♦ The aim of treatment is to produce a therapeutic response, and normally there is a range of serum concentrations that will produce such a response.
♦ The minimum effective concentration is at the lower end of this range and any concentration below this is said to be subtherapeutic.
♦ Above the top end of this range, the dose becomes toxic.
♦ The range in the middle where the concentration is therapeutic is called the therapeutic index or window.

Loading Doses

If a fast response is needed, then a loading dose can be used to bring the serum concentration to within the therapeutic levels after a single dose. Subsequent doses will then keep the drug at steady state. These doses may be calculated individually for patients or more commonly a standard loading dose will be given.

Examples

Digoxin given orally as a loading dose in atrial fibrillation or flutter is prescribed as a single dose of 0.75-1.5mg. If there is an increased risk of adverse effects (e.g. in the elderly) or reduced urgency in treatment then the dose can be divided and given six hours apart (See the SPC for digoxin and the BNF for further information).

Teicoplanin is a glycopeptide antibiotic used in gram positive infections. It is administered either intravenously or intramuscularly. Loading doses are given to bring serum levels in to therapeutic range. The first three doses are therefore loading doses and are given twelve hours apart. Further doses are then given every twenty-four hours.

Therapeutic Drug Monitoring (TDM)

Figure 4.14 highlights the concept that in practice, ideally we want to prescribe drugs where the therapeutic window is wide and the peak effects are well below the top end of the therapeutic window. What this means is that the range of concentrations that produce a therapeutic effect is wide enough to allow a wide safety margin when doses are given between both toxic and subtherapeutic concentrations. The reason for this is because individuals process drugs in different ways and so the same dose of a drug given to different people may well not lead to equivalent serum concentrations. If the range of therapeutic concentrations is narrow, then there is a real risk of a problem occurring in patients.

Most drugs have a relatively broad therapeutic window and so changes in serum concentration produced by licensed doses do not have a clinically significant impact (see **Figure 4.14**). There are some drugs that have a narrow therapeutic window, meaning that relatively small changes in serum concentration can lead to clinical impact. This may

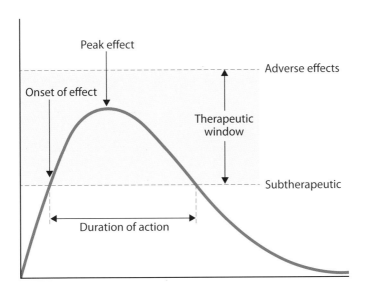

Figure 4.14 – Graph illustrating the therapeutic window

be a loss of therapeutic control on the one hand or toxicity on the other. These drugs are used because they are so effective for the conditions for which they are prescribed. However, the risk to patients is minimised for this group of drugs by monitoring serum levels. Most NHS Trusts and Clinical Commissioning Groups (CCGs) will have policies and guidelines on TDM – make sure you know where to access your local guidance.

Examples of drugs with a narrow therapeutic index are:

♦ Phenytoin
♦ Gentamicin
♦ Carbamazepine
♦ Digoxin
♦ Lithium
♦ Vancomycin
♦ Theophylline
♦ Ciclosporin

Key Points

♦ Time is taken for drug levels to reach steady state after repeated administration.
♦ Different doses will lead to different steady state levels, which may or may not be within the therapeutic window.
♦ For drugs that undergo zero order elimination at higher doses, steady state is not reached as there can be no equilibrium between absorption/elimination as the elimination system is saturated

Conclusion

In this chapter we have covered a range of concepts that you can use to help interpret information about the drugs you will be prescribing. Further reading is given below, with references to specific pharmacology textbooks which will give more detail on what has been covered. There are also links to websites which provide more information on drugs in practice. It is through exploring these resources, along with the local and national guidance, that you can build up your pharmacological knowledge and experience of the drugs that you will be working with. It may be useful to compile a personal formulary of drugs that you will be encountering, noting the key pharmacological aspects of these drugs.

Key Points of This Chapter

♦ Pharmacology is essential in understanding the mechanism of how drugs work and interact with the body.

♦ The concepts in this chapter can be applied to drugs you encounter in practice to enable you to be a safe and effective prescriber, though it will take time to build up knowledge and experience in your area of practice.

♦ Drugs act on targets in the body to produce some kind of physiological change.

♦ We can broadly group drugs in to agonists and antagonists.

♦ Remember pharmacokinetic parameters using ADME – absorption, distribution, metabolism and elimination.

♦ Be cautious when changing therapy in patients when parameters such as bioavailability, therapeutic index or CYP450 metabolism may be affected.

References and Further Reading

Burton, M.E., Shaw, L.M., Schentag, J.J. and Evans, W.E. (2006). *Applied Pharmacokinetics and Pharmacodynamics: Principles of Therapeutic Drug Monitoring*. Lippincott Williams & Wilkins, Baltimore.

Gard, P. (2001). *Human Pharmacology*. London: CRC Press.

Katzung, B., Masters, S. and Trevor, A. (eds) (2012). *Basic and Clinical Pharmacology*. Maidenhead: McGraw-Hill.

Kenakin, T.P. (2017). *Pharmacology in Drug Discovery and Development: Understanding drug response*. Oxford: Elsevier/Academic Press.

Koup, J. (1989). Disease states and drug pharmacokinetics. *Journal of Clinical Pharmacology* 29: 674–679.

Rang, H.P., Ritter, J.M., Flower, R.J. and Henderson, G. (2016). *Rang & Dale's Pharmacology*. Oxford: Elsevier/Churchill Livingstone.

Rosenbaum, D.M., Rasmussen, S.G.F. and Kobilka, B.K. (2009). The structure and function of G-protein coupled receptors. *Nature* 459(7245): 356–363.

Walker R., Whittlesea C. (eds) (2012). *Clinical Pharmacy and Therapeutics*. Oxford: Elsevier/Churchill Livingstone. (In particular Chapter 3 entitled practical pharmacokinetics).

Useful Websites

British National Formulary. This is the go to reference for individual medicines and will give you brief information on anything important linked to prescribing that medicine. Available at: https://bnf.nice.org.uk.

The Electronic Medicines Compendium (eMC) is a database of the SPCs for medicines that are licensed in the UK. The SPC contains more detailed information than the BNF entries and is useful to refer to for learning and when you have a more complex patient. It has specific sections that cover the pharmacological properties of licensed medicines. Available at: https://www.medicines.org.uk/emc.

The National Institute for Clinical Excellence (NICE) includes guidance on various topics, such as managing ADRs, prescribing in renal disease. It is important to be aware of what guidance they have that may influence your practice as they are a national NHS body producing evidence based guidance. Available at: https://www.nice.org.uk.

NHS Specialist Pharmacy Services (SPS) is a website that has useful information on prescribing for staff working in the NHS. There are various articles that review evidence and aim to help prescribing decisions, particularly where there is limited evidence. Available at: https://www.sps.nhs.uk.

The online version of the Merck Manuals has a section on clinical pharmacology that you may find useful for general background info on pharmacological concepts: https://www.msdmanuals.com/professional/clinical-pharmacology.

Chapter 5
Decision Making for Prescribing
Andy Collen

In This Chapter

- Introduction
- An overview of decision making
- Decision-making models
- Human factors in decision making
- Professional insight
- The practical application of decision-making theory to prescribing practice
- Principles of best practice in prescribing
- Key points of the chapter
- References

Introduction

This chapter will look at the theoretical models which exist in practice and provide or reinforce the cognitive processing acumen needed, particularly by prescribers, to logically and safely provide care for patients. It will look primarily at hypothetic-deduction, as this is the common approach of medical decision making, and how its component parts can promote better accuracy. The topic of human factors will also be reviewed and will include an overview of the cognitive biases which should be considered when trying to arrive at a diagnosis for a patient.

An important theme that runs throughout this chapter and the wider decision-making literature, and is included in the raft of reports on errors made by humans over the last three or four decades in healthcare and other safety-critical industries such as aviation is professional insight.

The chapter concludes by stating the principles of good prescribing, 'best practice' and provides some useful 'mnemonics' and asks readers to consider a case study.

The prescribing pyramid and the competency framework for all prescribers that are introduced in **Chapter 3** are referred to in this chapter with particular reference to the decision-making process and relevant theory.

An Overview of Decision Making

Human beings make decisions constantly, most of which are done without conscious thought or consideration. Those which do require more thought often happen quickly and with minimal additional active processing. We are able to accumulate experiences and use these as 'stored procedures', called heuristics, which allow us to operate in our daily lives without having to actually think about everything we do. The acquisition of experience (practice) and using this experience (skill) can help us get better at what we do (expertise). Consider how a child approaches the building of a new Lego model – slowly and deliberately following the instructions, page by page, until it is completed. After a few times of rebuilding the same model, and depending on its complexity, the instructions may become redundant and the speed of the build reduces. In adult life we do this too; this is helpful in the mastery of activities such as sports and playing musical instruments, but less helpful where we try to make more complex decisions in dynamic and challenging contexts (as we do in healthcare). There is a fundamental concept that all humans need to accept, and that is that we are not cognitively perfect or elegant – far from it, we are in actual fact positively flawed in terms of how we perceive, process and store information. We are prone to making errors where we fail to appreciate these flaws and accept how they limit us. In recent years, this realisation (and growing acceptance) has crystallised under the banner of the 'Human Factors' movement, the study of how the human condition has an effect on the activities we undertake. Appreciating that 'though we cannot change the human condition, we can change the conditions under which humans work' (Reason, 2000, p. 768), we can improve what we do and how we do it: firstly, by appreciating the magnitude of the challenges; and, secondly, by seeking strategies to improve our decision-making acumen. Some of the principles of resolving human factors are intrinsic (how the person approaches the issue) and some are extrinsic (how humans improve the design of things we use), and irrespective of the various domains of human factors, it requires insight and humility in order to embrace these frailties. No one wants to be accept that they are bad at something they have been doing for many years. The subtle shift from a fixed mindset ('I have a fixed amount of talent and ability') to a growth mindset ('I can always improve and grow') (Dweck, 2006) suggests that in clinical practice we need continually improve and focus on quality as a way of promoting safe and effective patient care.

The nub of the problem for us as a species is that we have evolved very significantly over millennia to the point where we are cognitively functional at a level beyond any other species, as evidenced by our ability to use language and our other higher mental functions. This development in our brains' abilities, while extremely useful, is affected anatomically by being made up from three distinct parts which combined throughout our evolutionary history, but never fully integrated. The human brain as we know it now had humble beginnings in the creatures which existed at the time before leaving the water to move on to the land. These initially tiny organs were located structurally at one end of an emerging nervous system, forming behind the eyes of those creatures from which mammalian life eventually developed (Robson, 2011). This 'lizard brain' was joined over millions of years by the evolving mammalian brain (the cerebellum) and eventually the bigger, more complex 'human bit' (the cerebrum) which made the brain larger overall. As well as being able to control the body in response to stimuli in a primitive way, it was able to make more judgements. In humans, the lizard brain remained and continued to evolve, and is now responsible for aspects of personality, mood and addiction, but started off controlling much more basic functions used to promote survival (fear, fight, flight, feeding, freezing, fornicate). It is this part of our brains which causes us problems with decision making. Linked to these distinct parts of our brains, and how they function, the Nobel Prize winner Daniel Kahneman described the two types of thinking:

♦   system 1 – fast and unconscious; and
♦   system 2 – slow and deliberate (Kahneman, 2011).

It is the system 1 part of our brain, which originates within the limbic system, which is at odds with our human brain, which is capable of system 2 thinking.

Decision making in clinical practice is fraught with risks and issues for the clinician. Understanding how to make decisions is only one consideration within the overall approach to safe and effective patient care and which is also enjoyable for the clinician to undertake (remembering that working under stress/duress reduces cognitive bandwidth due to the release of stress hormones which leads to 'lizard-like' behaviours, namely fight/flight). Understanding that we can be misled by the oldest parts of our brain, learning to distrust it and allow ourselves time to overcome this impediment can make us much safer in practice. This can also engender more professional insight and a desire to promote a continuum of learning – developing a scientific approach to what you experience in practice; deducing more and assuming less.

Expanding practice to include prescribing requires a very well-developed sense of ability and limitation. Medicines, once administered or taken, cannot be ungiven and this means that diagnostic accuracy, care planning and aftercare must be right every time. The decisions which guide prescribing are exponentially more complex due to the considerations of how diseases intersect with therapy in the presence of patient variation, allergies, interactions and the other myriad complexities which must be approached with reverence. Practice that is led only by experientially derived intuition, compared to practice that is approached scientifically and rigorously, differs only in terms of the regard given to the patient, their outcomes and their safety.

Theoretical Models

Decision making is a human task or endeavour rather than an aspect of clinical care. In healthcare, the term 'clinical decision making' is commonly used and suggests that we make decisions differently in practice compared to our everyday life. Challenging this and using good structured decision-making skills in other parts of your life provide opportunities to hone your deductive skills and challenge yourself to avoid the pitfalls of the human condition. Clearly, this does not mean becoming a robot and missing out on the spontaneous decisions which make life enjoyable, such as making an impulse purchase or having that one last drink which leads to a worse hangover. However, a good decision maker can enhance their everyday life as well as their professional life by refining their skills and speeding up the process to good decisions, and leading to less situations involving regret ('I wish I hadn't bought that car, the boot just isn't big enough').

The different theoretical models which exist are either intuition-based (gestalt) or use some kind of scientific process. Arguably, pure intuition in diagnostic (as opposed to humanist) healthcare is inappropriate. While a 'gut-feeling' gives healthcare professionals the insight to know that a patient is upset or in pain, it is not sufficient to rule in or out serious diseases, particularly where the decision is apparently obvious. Harm in healthcare often occurs where consideration is not given to that which is rare or unlikely. This links to the biases and 'shortcuts' we use as humans in everyday life. Where there are competing options or theories, the application of 'Occam's Razor' can be helpful as a principle which can drive yourself to challenge your thinking – choose the option which requires the least assumptions (Hamilton, 1862). In other words, if it feels correct, make sure it does not have any baggage or require a leap of faith. For example, the diagnosis is fine if the patient's acute illness is the only illness they have and they do not have another disease process that could be masking or skewing the convenient (and potentially biased) diagnosis given.

Any decision-making model which relies on any form or scientific enquiry rather than only a gut-feeling or intuition is essentially hypothetico-deductive – in simple terms, the development of a list of theories (hypotheses) which need to be tested and/or potentially retested to reach (deduce) a conclusion for each of these theories or hypotheses, and then whittling these down to a smaller number (or even a single) diagnosis which can evidentially be addressed via a definitive therapeutic process or be referred on for further enquiry. Patients rarely present in previously perfect health and with a condition that can be conveniently identified as truly definitive. In reality, there has to be room for ambiguity and which is turn means that any element of risk will be present, and this reinforces the importance of providing clear advice for patients following their encounter. Importantly for clinicians, such as paramedics, who often work in a scientifically austere environments and who rely on clinical assessment, there should be no pressure or expectation to reach the end point of the deductive or therapeutic process. It is not a failure to reach a point where further enquiry is needed (for example, sending the patient to hospital for an x-ray), and reaching the line of capability where the number of hypotheses cannot be further reduced will lead to a further decision in itself – to refer the patient on (see **Figure 5.1**). In the context of prescribing, this reinforces the decision to not prescribe where appropriate and the need to ensure that the pressure to prescribe is controlled.

An aspect of decision making that cannot be overlooked is the requirement to have sound clinical knowledge and competency within the scope of the clinician's practice, and the experience of seeing the conditions that the paramedic is expecting to prescribe for. The hypothesis generation required in order to deduce the diagnosis requires clinical expertise and a level of artistry in practice commensurate to the magnitude of the clinical situation. Paramedics rarely undertake truly specialised practice and are in many ways 'extended generalists' or 'expert generalists' (Benner, 1984). This creates additional challenges when working in urgent and emergency care settings where patients present throughout the age spectrum and across the cornucopia of diseases.

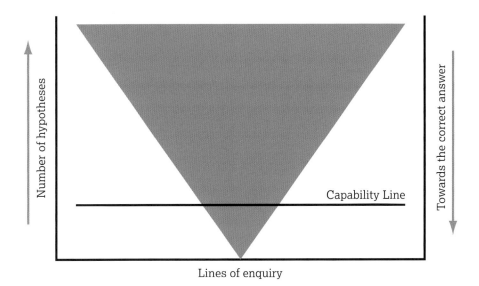

Figure 5.1 – Line of capability

To make a decision or judgement, first you need information and evidence to review. This information must be of good quality and you must be capable of appraising it, and assessing its provenance and suitability. There are two important skills associated with the gathering of information, critical thinking and information processing. Information processing (as a component of hypothetico-deduction) is the act of quality controlling and challenging the information. After this, critical thinking can be applied as a way of considering the information – applying a level of scepticism to appropriately validate what it is you are seeing, being told, measuring and so on. For example, how would you critically appraise the following pieces of information?:

♦ 65-year-old male
♦ Five-day history of abdominal pain
♦ Has not passed urine for three days
♦ Has not had his bowels open for five days
♦ Has not eaten for seven days.

There is a great temptation to leap to a diagnosis which may, or perhaps may not, appear obvious, maybe leaning towards a bowel obstruction. The 'elephant in the room' for decision makers is that most of the time, your gut feeling or intuition is accurate, but that would be a judgement based on hindsight. On occasions, when your intuition is incorrect, hindsight will provide no defence to the clinician or comfort for a patient or their family. Looking back at the list of information and looking at it in a truly critical way, you may formulate other questions to satisfy yourself that it is correct. This does not have to be onerous and can be done through further brief questioning and reinforcement. For example:

- 65-year-old male ('What is your date of birth?' ... 'You're actually 75!')
- Five-day history of abdominal pain ('Point to where it hurts' ... 'So more in your back then?')
- Has not passed urine for three days ('You can still pass a trickle, you say?' ... 'The patient is making urine')
- Has not had his bowels open for five days (Patient: 'it's not a proper movement – quite watery' ... 'Have you actually passed a stool?')
- Has not eaten for seven days (Patient: 'not proper meals, just snacking').

In much the same way that clinicians are fallible as human beings, so are patients and the data they produce (either verbally or as signs which may not fit a 'classic' or textbook definition of the diseases they represent). The information they provide is often imprecise, inaccurate, subjective, emotionally influenced, guarded, omitted, skewed, biased and, on occasion, false. The skill of critically analysing the information you receive from the patient and ranking it in terms of importance and relevance is vital. Of course, this extends to what you elicit from them in your physical examination and physiological measurement – the approach to which is honed in practice, focusing on the investigations most likely to yield a finding (for example, confirming adventitia upon auscultation). A common example is where patients report a pain score of 10 out of 10, but they are not outwardly distressed, sweaty, tachycardic or showing any other classic signs of exquisite pain. Of course, 'pain is what the patient says it is' (McCaffery, 1968), but this must be balanced against the ethical requirement to do only what is of benefit to the patient (beneficence) and minimising the risk of harm when considering treatment (non-maleficence) (Beauchamp and Childress, 2001). In a prescribing context, this may lead to a more conservative approach to analgesia, for example.

There are barriers to critical thinking which can prevent enquiry, and which are often deeply embedded (unconscious bias). These include sociocentricity ('group-think'), egocentricity (self-belief in own beliefs), selfishness (lack of consideration for patient), desire for wish fulfilment (wanting to believe things, even if they are wrong) and self-validation ('I have always done it this way', with an unwillingness to change). These concepts are challenging for a variety of reasons and require very significant personal insight, humility and courage. These traits are those of effective people. The transition to becoming a prescriber has to include personal development to ensure that decisions are made with due consideration to these factors and influences. There are many other, sometimes more subtle, barriers to critical thinking, such as conformism, denial, comfort zones and cognitive dissonance, all of which conspire to affect the way information is perceived and processed. Understanding these is a crucial aspect of taming the human condition and becoming a more effective decision maker.

 Turn to **Chapter 10** for more information about personal reflection and professional development.

Using information processing and critical thinking side by side is a helpful way of ensuring that when you begin to undertake the actual deductive process that will take you towards your diagnosis or other end-point decision, the information will be optimised and "quality assured". It will contribute to the reduction in the impact of an erroneous pieces of information which may contaminate the overall process. Bearing in mind that patients are complex, disease processes often mimic one another, and the practical application is not as straightforward as it sounds. It will be tempting to continue to use only your experience and intuition, which is fine if this extends only to generating high-quality hypotheses!

Hypothesis generation is little more than a list of things that it could be (an educated guess or differential diagnoses). A patient with central chest pain could have one or more of a number of diseases, some of which are rare and some of which are common. It is worth noting at this point that in the case of a true medical emergency, you cannot spend long periods of time ensuring that you have the correct diagnosis. Instead, you must prepare for the worst, based on the chief complaint. This is called 'shot-gunning' (Klein et al., 1993) and uses the 'obvious' to drive the 'essential'. For patients whose disease process can be managed on a slower care continuum, perhaps with a five or six-day history of continuous chest pain with no other 'classic' cardiac signs or symptoms, the creation of the list of hypotheses (differential diagnoses) will still include myocardial infarction, but this may be lower down the clinician's index of suspicion. As the decision maker improves their acumen, the list of hypotheses may be formed more quickly and be more refined compared to the novice. This may be based on examples in practice or domain knowledge. To give an obvious example, abdominal pain in patients without a uterus/ovaries is very unlikely to be a complication of pregnancy. It is an important point for the novice (and in particular those becoming prescribers) that the ability to create effective hypotheses is unaffected by experience. While the list may be longer than those further along Benner's 'novice to expert' journey (Benner, 1984), the evidence suggests that hypothesis generation has similar accuracy.

Once you have ruled out the most urgent problems (requiring rapid action or 'shot-gunning') and have formed a list of differential diagnoses, you need to test these hypotheses in order to deduce the answer, hence the term 'hypothetico-deduction'. The actual process of deduction uses a range of techniques on a gradient or 'cognitive continuum' (Hamm, 1988), which varies according to mode and reliability. In Figure 5.2, you can see that intuition is at the opposite end of the spectrum from scientific experimentation and is considered 'ill structured', whereas scientific experiment is well structured and analytical. Clearly it is unrealistic to discover new knowledge about a patient using controlled trials (mode 2) and scientific experiment (mode 1) in everyday clinical practice, nor is it appropriate to use only intuitive judgements to resolve every practice dilemma. The cognitive continuum suggests a fluid state, moving around the differing modes to help test each hypothesis. As an example and in the context of medicines and prescribing, when selecting the correct drug to prescribe, you are unlikely to guess or use intuition; rather, you would look up the correct drug, dose, presentation, etc. in the BNF or local prescribing guidance (mode 4) and may even discuss the options with a colleague (mode 5).

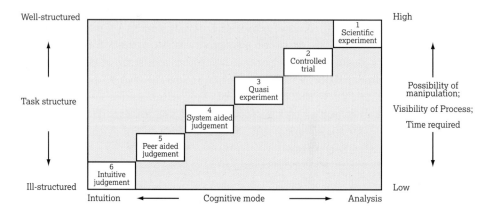

Figure 5.2 – The cognitive continuum

Source: Hamm, R. (1988). Clinical Intuition and clinical analysis: expertise and the cognitive continuum. In J. Dowie and A. Eisten (eds), *Professional Judgement: A reader in clinical decision making.* Cambridge: Cambridge University Press.

When working through the list of hypotheses, the same approach is true and may include quasi-experimentation (mode 3) in the form of physiological measurements (blood pressure, ECG, urinalysis). This would almost certainly include referring to the evidence based which is developed using controlled trials (mode 2). The most common system-aided judgement tool in healthcare practice is clinical practice guidance – for example, the NICE Guidelines (NICE, 2018). Electronic decision support tools and software are also becoming more common, and undoubtedly artificial intelligence (AI) will play an increasing role in healthcare in the future, but mindful that the process of diagnosis almost always requires human interactions in form of negotiation, building trust, and the other aspects of human enterprise to achieve the outcome which can form a contract of care. A machine may never be capable of achieving this level of ability, and may only serve to support human decision makers

The demand on health services and the call on clinicians' time is becoming ever more challenging. This can lead to a pressure to work more quickly and potentially in more isolation. On the basis that 'no man [or woman] is an island', clinicians and in particular those making complex decisions, such as whether to prescribe, must be very aware of these pressures and must strive to minimise the risks of working in isolation by sharing some decisions, both with patients and with colleagues. There is little to be gained by priding oneself in doing everything on one's own and trying to get it right without any help. Conversely, there is much to lose by causing avoidable harm to a patient because of a misplaced or stubborn need to validate one's practice by practising in isolation and without the professional insight needed when dealing with undifferentiated care. When considering collaborating and sharing decisions, the clinician with primacy of care retains professional responsibility and the temptation to abdicate responsibility must be avoided. The difference between spreading cognitive load and passing on responsibility may be subtle and should be understood by all parties involved.

In some care settings, the patients are obviously extremely ill and while this is extremely challenging healthcare, it is unlikely that the patient will be discharged in error while being profoundly unconscious due to a cerebral haemorrhage. In urgent care settings, where patients often present on the basis of wanting to resolve symptoms which they believe involve nothing sinister, there is the ever-present risk of missing something very serious. Deciding to prescribe based only on palliating symptoms in a patient with an acute but apparently benign presentation suggests a poor decision-making process and is arguably most likely to result from an intuitive assumption. Remember the reference to Occam's Razor (Hamilton, 1862): choose the option that requires the fewest assumptions. Assuming every patient with a headache simply has a generalised headache without further enquiry, thus adding more assumptions, is not safe or appropriate. For example, you may assume that every patient with a thunderclap headache has a bleed. Conversely, for patients who present with a thunderclap headache but have a history of migraine, you may assume the migraine is the cause of the headache. Migraineurs are at no greater risk of having a cerebral bleed but may be overlooked due to their history of headache.

In summarising this section, the actual application of hypothetico-deduction is relatively straightforward and certainly well within the cognitive bandwidth of a clinician considering expanding their practice to include prescribing. The problem with decision making is the constant bombardment of distractions, competing priorities, stress, hunger, fatigue and the other myriad factors which can fill one's bandwidth and cognitive capacity beyond its functional range. If understood, this can be controlled. Therefore, understanding 'human factors' is an essential component in the decision makers' toolkit.

Human Factors

We have already discussed why from an anatomical and evolutionary perspective the human condition has become what it is and how this can cause a range of problems. It is becoming increasingly unpopular to compare the aviation industry to healthcare in terms of how managing human factors can change outcomes. But it cannot be overlooked that in 2017, there was not a single fatality resulting from an accident involving a commercial passenger aircraft and, in the UK, there has not been a passenger fatality since 1999 (Aviation Safety Network, 2018). These statistics are a reflection of a focus on the way aviation approached the errors resulting from the human condition in the industry and considers the fact that planes rarely catastrophically fail. Accidents are almost always down to 'human error'. It is the focus on resolving the conditions that the humans (pilots) work in that has changed the landscape of commercial aviation and its enviable safety record in the modern age. In healthcare in the UK, consistently, year on year, it is estimated that around 9,000 patients die as a result of avoidable errors (Department of Health and Social Care, 2017). In aviation terms, that would equate to a plane crashing every day and resulting in the death of every passenger on board. Critics argue that airline passengers arrive at the airport in good health and go from healthy and happy to dead very suddenly, due only to the trauma of crashing. Conversely, patients arrive at the healthcare facility in poor condition and therefore any unexpected demise is more likely due to this pre-existing reduction in health. While this is true of very sick people presenting to an emergency department and being admitted to an intensive therapy unit (ITU), patients presenting with an apparently minor problems, or who are having an elective procedure, should not expect to die. Their families would not excuse any errors on the basis that they were already ill. In many ways the fact that patients are already vulnerable and less able to tolerate an error should focus healthcare systems more, rather than excuse those errors citing the underlying frailty of patients.

Therefore, while aviation analogies may have become tiresome for some, the principles regarding how the aviation industry addressed the things that were killing its passengers were successful and can be transferred to other industries, including healthcare.

Human factors is a very wide topic and covers concepts such as ergonomics, design, communication, environment, team dynamics, cognition, workload, fatigue… and the list goes on. In the context of decision making in the diagnostic and therapy planning paradigm, arguably the most important human factors which negatively influence outcomes are cognitive biases. The other human factors are extremely important, particularly communication. The reader is advised to look at sources of information on the wider topic of human factors produced by the Clinical Human Factors Group (https://chfg.org). The group was set up by airline captain Martin Bromiley, whose wife sadly died during the anaesthetic phase of an elective operation. His courage in the face of this tragedy should not be overlooked. The film produced by the group 'Just a Routine Operation' encompasses the litany of issues which led to Elaine Bromiley's avoidable death from a hypoxic brain injury. You can find the film by searching in Google or YouTube using the search term 'just a routine operation'. The ongoing role of the Clinical Human Factors Group is to:

♦ Design for safety. Embed Human Factors science into procurement, design and delivery of care.
♦ Learn from success and failure. Encourage a just culture, better local investigations, so mistakes are not repeated and success is.
♦ Educate and promote Human Factors in all healthcare settings.
(Clinical Human Factors Group, 2018)

Learning from incidents and errors is an essential part of healthcare and has been part of aviation for many decades. In his book *Black Box Thinking*, Matthew Syed (2015) describes how the use of data analysis following an incident can provide insight into prevention. In healthcare this translates into the professional activities that clinicians must engage in; continuing professional development, supervision, audit, debrief, mortality and morbidity review, and reflection.

 Turn to **Chapter 10** for more details on some of the topics mentioned above.

Returning to the focus on cognitive biases, clinicians (and all decision makers in safety-critical systems) need to develop vigilance towards their own negative influences. There are around 100 biases and fallacies which affect humans and are usually highly illogical. The problem we suffer from is the way we automatically process, store and recall information in our long-term and short-term memories, and how these factors affect other memories and beliefs, particularly in high-pressure situations. An example of where people in stressful situations record a memory and recall it with certainty is after witnessing a crime. The police will often record wildly different accounts from people who witness an armed robbery taking place, who contradict each other in terms of the number of robbers, the clothes they were wearing, the vehicles they used and the direction they escaped in. This is an example of where the brain is taken over by the old part of the brain in response to danger and how this diminishes the higher functions, effectively reducing the bandwidth and pixelating the images or adding or removing details. A famous example of this is the assassination of President Kennedy in November 1963. Witnesses reported anything between two and eight gunshots coming from the Texas School Book Depository, the Daltex Building, the Grassy Knoll and the Triple Overpass at the end of Dealey Plaza. Some reported seeing muzzle flashes and smoke, and many reported smelling cordite (the chemical used in ammunition). The overwhelming emotional response to watching the President of the United States being shot significantly reduced the witnesses' usefulness and ultimately prevented any enduringly meaningful conclusion being drawn on the assassination.

With this in mind, what have we seen in the past that we have stored as a fact and recalled incorrectly, such as remembering a family party where we recalled that a particular person was there, but in fact they could not have been (i.e. they were out of the country). They probably had been at another event and the two events become 'stitched together' for the brain's convenience, and this becomes the most available thought. Availability bias is one of the common biases seen in human psychology and is the brain's way of exploiting its own innate laziness by allowing that which is easy or nearby to influence the decision, either mentally as ideation or practically (perhaps by choosing not to use a piece of equipment which may refute a theory). Another very important bias in healthcare is conjunction, which is where there is a lack of appreciation that two things can happen at once. For example, the patient who comes home from a foreign holiday with very obvious cellulitis may also have a deep vein thrombosis (DVT). While this is unlikely, the overwhelmingly unequivocal diagnosis of cellulitis can erroneously mark the end of the diagnostic process, rather than truly exploring the differential diagnoses, which must include DVT. Conjunction may exist in parallel with confirmation bias and using the previous example, the confirmatory stimuli relating to the cellulitis (classic history, evidence of wound, demarcation, spread, fever) 'drowns out' the other parts of the clinical picture, which become ignored. The signs and symptoms (and history) relating to the risk of DVT are still there; they do not cease to exist just because they are being disregarded. In an era of ever-increasing co-morbidity and multi-morbidity in our increasingly ageing population, the chances of finding multiple acute disease processes may be overlooked, but can lead to tragic and catastrophic outcomes for patients and their families.

The list of biases is very long and cannot be covered in this short section, and you should explore them in more detail in other sources (Collen, 2017). There is one final bias which is worth highlighting, as it may affect professions such as paramedics more than others. Action bias is the drive and desire to do something, and is linked to the deontological approach that emergency care providers often have. In some cases the outcome is judged on the overall intention to do 'good', such as we see with futile resuscitation attempts. For prescribers, the urge to prescribe needs to be controlled as the overall 'good' may in fact be derived from not prescribing or, indeed, de-prescribing. In some practice settings, patients may present with very clear expectations of the outcome; this may include specific requests for antibiotics or other named medicines. There are two concepts which need to be considered by the decision maker where action bias needs to be controlled: antimicrobial resistance and substance misuse. Antimicrobial resistance is likely to be the greatest challenge for healthcare in the modern age. While the established oral antibiotics are less emphasised in the impact of growing resistance (compared to the broad-spectrum intravenous antibiotics), the concept of 'antimicrobial stewardship' should guide practice, and the decision to prescribe these medicines in response to the desire to act needs to be carried out with a clear rationale. In many ways, the second consideration – substance misuse or dependence – may be even more challenging for paramedics in a prescribing role, particularly in community settings. At the point when the law changed to allow paramedic prescribing (the amendment of the Human Medicines Regulation on 1 April 2018), this did not include the ability to prescribe controlled drugs. Part of the consultation to introduce independent prescribing included seeking support for the legal authority to prescribe from a limited formulary of controlled drugs. Prescribing of these medicines can only happen once the Misuse of Drugs regulations is amended to reflect these additional responsibilities. There is greater emphasis on medicines dependency and misuse, and the paramedic making decisions in future about the prescribing of CDs needs to consider patients at risk of these issues. Patients suffering dependence on prescribed medicines, or those who seek to misuse medicines, will often approach multiple health facilities to obtain multiple prescriptions. Paramedics may find themselves practising in the kinds of facilities where these patients present (for example, out-of-hours providers and emergency departments) and therefore should be aware of, and vigilant towards, these risks and control any bias towards action. Those seeking to obtain medicines for misuse or dependence may ask for medicines by name. They may also provide false information and clinical symptoms. The action bias should become an intrinsic consideration for decision makers alongside all the other human factors and cognitive biases and barriers we are subject to.

 Turn to **Chapter 2** for more on the legal and ethical aspects of prescribing, and to **Chapter 7** to read more about the public health issues of prescribing.

The primary reason for making good decisions is patient safety. The clinician owes a professional, moral and ethical duty to the patient to do no harm (non-maleficence) and to do only that which provides the patient with a benefit (beneficence) (Beauchamp and Childress, 2001). In many aspects of life, hindsight is a wonderful thing, but in healthcare it is not, regardless of the outcome – good or bad. Clinical practice should be a joy and undertaken without being permanently crippled by fear, and while learning from error is part of reflective practice and continuous improvement and development, the fundamental principle to do no harm must drive care – mindful that we are not going to get it right every time, and that risk management and mitigation is part of the decision making process. By linking your knowledge of human factors and directing the challenges that this brings (such as increasing your humility and reducing your ego) towards patient safety, the chances of being a victim of hindsight are reduced. It is never good to hear in a Coroner's Court that, in hindsight, the patient also had DVT as well as cellulitis.

Human factors in healthcare are better understood now than ever before. Clinicians should continue to aspire to the levels of understanding and professional insight that transformed commercial aviation, mindful that operating a machine (aircraft) is different to providing care to patients, but the haptic feedback a pilot feels through the controls may be compared to experience of a patient encounter in terms of its ever changing and sometimes unpredictable dynamic. Considering all of the aspects of the human condition that negatively affect decision making is important, but it is also important to remember that healthcare involves risks. It is the mitigation of these risks rather than avoidance of risk which improves care. A well-developed decision-making acumen is essential for prescribers, and while the novice phase of mastering hypothetico-deduction may feel clumsy (akin to watching a toddler taking their first deliberate and uncoordinated steps), the fluency will come and become a natural part of your practice. Making prescribing more satisfying for you and safer for your patients.

The Practical Application of Decision Making in Prescribing Practice

Decision making is woven through all aspects of clinical practice, and will extend to your prescribing practice too. As discussed previously, 'prescribing' may involve very little actual prescribing. It is therefore perhaps more accurate to describe the role of a non-medical prescriber as a truly holistic clinician who can apply the principles and competence intrinsic to prescribing throughout the patient's journey, from the point at which the patient first presents to the end point of care and beyond if necessary. The moment in time when the prescriber puts pen to paper (or fingers to keyboard) to actually prescribe a new medicine is the end of a detailed and complex decision-making journey, the destination point of which carries perhaps the most consequence and significance.

Paramedics are fortunate in that by the time they begin to introduce prescribing into their practice, they will have had many years of experience of providing care and treatment involving medicines. The addition of prescribing to the existing medicines mechanisms that paramedics have serves to remind the paramedic of one of the most important factors when supplying or administering medicines: once taken or administered, medicines cannot be 'ungiven' (although some may be antagonised). It is this consequence that is amplified for prescribers and therefore requires the most accurate and effective decisions to be made. It is also the case that many of the drugs that paramedics are able to administer in an emergency have limited long-term physiological consequences, even where dosing errors occur (acute complications, such as respiratory depression associated with benzodiazepines and opiates, require urgent intervention, but are unlikely to cause long-term harm if correctly managed). Even the supply of short courses of analgesia or antibiotics under a PGD has relatively limited consequences, such as the classic 'howlers' of giving amoxicillin to patients with glandular fever, which is unpleasant and unsightly but not dangerous. Other errors will have far greater consequences. Some will result from diagnostic errors and some from human errors, such as the simple muddling of drug names. If not noticed at the point of dispensing, this may prove to be catastrophic. For example, if you are not aware of your own level of fatigue or other pressures of work, similar-looking words can be mistaken. For example, if the last patient you saw was prescribed ranitidine for their gastric ulcer, this could be written on the next patient's prescription instead of rivaroxaban. This could be much worse if the order was reversed, and therefore good information processing is essential.

Thinking back to the previous part of this chapter, perhaps the most important aspect of the practical aspect of decision making is deciding that the medicines proposed for prescribing are correct. Beyond using good decision making to avoid harm and error and to reach the diagnosis (or alternative if a diagnosis is not possible, such as referral), the cognitive continuum may continue into the selection of the medicine you are going to prescribe. Alternatively, it might lead to the decision not to prescribe or to change the patient's existing medicines regimen (including de-prescribing).

The core prescribing curriculum will provide the knowledge and skills to become a competent prescriber and meet the individual competencies, which bring together the tenets for safe, patient centred prescribing. The use of shared decision making and building the relationship between clinician and patient, with the aim of reaching common care goals, is an essential aspect of the overall decision-making process. Patients may approach their needs with very clear goals or with limited expectations beyond simply getting better. Some patients become experts in their own long-term diseases and can assist greatly in the decision-making process, obviously with due regard to the risk of dependency. For example, a patient with ulcerative colitis who experiences a flare-up of their symptoms may want a course of steroids or may suggest a change of route of administration from oral tablets to rectal foam for their mesalazine. Underpinning the importance of shared decision making among the other core components of the *Competency Framework for All Prescribers* (see **Figure 5.3**).

The decision-making skills that aspirant prescribers bring with them to their prescribing practice continue to develop and refine as part of their continuing professional development, and will be enhanced by the additional knowledge and skills which are included in their prescribing education and the ongoing supervision that prescribers undertake. Prescribing, in the main, is not protocol-driven and the use of guidance and judgement to drive practice is a significant step even for paramedics who practise at an advanced level. Embracing a hypothetico-deductive approach and/or its component

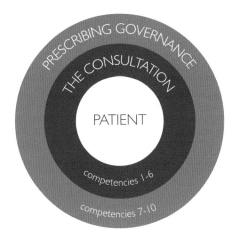

THE CONSULTATION	PRESCRIBING GOVERNANCE
1. Assess the patient	7. Prescribe safely
2. Consider the options	8. Prescribe professionally
3. Reach a shared decision	9. Improve prescribing practice
4. Prescribe	10. Prescribe as part of a team
5. Provide information	
6. Monitor and review	

Figure 5.3 – Competency Framework for All Prescribers

Source: Royal Pharmaceutical Society (2016). *The Competency Framework for All Prescribers*. London: Royal Pharmaceutical Society.

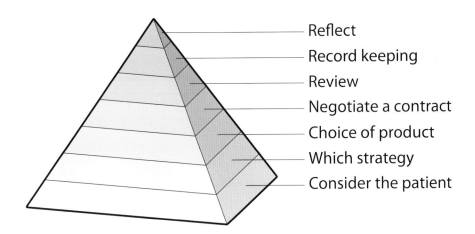

Figure 5.4 – The prescribing pyramid

Source: National Prescribing Centre (1999). *Nurse Prescribing Bulletin*. Signposts for prescribing nurses – general principles of good prescribing. London: National Prescribing Centre

parts (such as critical thinking) can be used to make better, safer decisions in all aspects of clinical practice, including prescribing. With the enhanced knowledge which comes with becoming a prescriber, the ability to appraise complex information about the diseases and medicines which are brought together in the treatment of patients can provide the clinician with the necessary skills to provide safe and effective patient care, which is arrived at robustly and systematically.

Principles of Good Prescribing

The principles of good prescribing is emphasised throughout this book, and the prescribing pyramid (see **Figure 5.4**) involves activities which requires effective cognitive processing and decision making. The Prescribing Pyramid is covered again in **Chapter 3** as part of the overarching consultation process.

Every level in the prescribing pyramid requires the processing of information and the development of a solution, approach, plan or consideration. Each point links to the decision-making principles discussed throughout this chapter and can be used to enhance the patient's experience of care, their safety, and the wellbeing of the clinician:

1. Consider the Patient

This involves the most fundamental question about whether the patient needs a prescription and whether the decision is made to not prescribe (or possibly de-prescribe). This is based on the decisions which arise from the history taking and assessment of the patient, and considers patient expectations and their safety (e.g. red flags, allergies).

2. Which Strategy?

Choosing the correct approach based on the wider consider of the patient's expectations is crucial to the success of the encounter. This includes consideration of the 'expert patient' who has very clear expectations and also the patient who is at risk of misuse or dependence. The strategy may be to refer on instead of treating definitively and involves the professional insight which prevents action bias and other factors that inhibit good decision making.

3. Choice of Product

Selecting the correct medicine is an absolutely critical decision and must consider a range of factors which can be remembered using the EASE mnemonic (see **Box 5.1**). You may have a personal formulary or be working as a supplementary prescriber, using a clinical management plan; regardless, you should ensure that you are familiar with the medicine being chosen. You should check the product's characteristics in the BNF to ensure that the patient's other medicines do not create interactions or other adverse reactions. In some practice settings, prescribers may be able to access decision support via the information technology (IT) system. For example, many primary care computer systems can be used to improve decisions and identify medicines which interact.

4. Negotiate a Contract

The principle of shared decision making between patient and clinician is vitally important in promoting the effective use of any medicines prescribed. There is little point prescribing a medicine if the patient stops taking it, and so working with the patient and communicating effectively will help them understand the importance of concordance in the resolution of their illness. You should discuss with the patient aspects of the treatment to ensure they can link their expectations accordingly – for example, explaining that the medicine will take several days to work before the patient experiences any change in their condition.

5. Review

Patients should be reviewed to ensure that the treatment given is effective and does not cause the patient any problems. For paramedics working in primary care settings, this may be done as part of an ongoing therapeutic relationship, but for those working in urgent care settings, follow-up and review may need to be arranged as part of any referral or discharge processes.

6. Record Keeping

Common to every aspect of professional healthcare provision, record keeping is of vital importance to ensure that a concise and accurate record of the patient's encounters is made.

7. Reflect

Prescribing is an ongoing professional journey and requires continual professional activities to support competency and confidence in practice. Reflecting on prescribing decisions is important and can ensure that those cognitive biases are better understood and future prescribing decisions are made. It is also necessary to decide on the follow-up and aftercare strategies, including worsening care advice and safety netting (there is more information on this in **Chapter 3**)

Mnemonics can be a useful way for prescribers to ensure that the key considerations are made for each clinical encounter. There are a wide variety of mnemonics available and these cover more than just the actual act of prescribing, taking on the history taking and physical assessment findings too (see **Box 5.1**).

Box 5.1 – Various mnemonics that the prescriber may find useful

EASE

E	How **effective** is the product?
A	Is it **appropriate**?
S	How **safe is** it?
E	Is the prescription cost **effective**?

SIT DOWN SIR

S	**Site** or location of a sign/symptom
I	**Intensity** or severity
T	**Type** or nature
D	**Duration**
O	**Onset**
W	**With** (other symptoms)
N	**Annoyed** or aggravated by
S	**Spread** or radiation
I	**Incidence** or frequency
R	**Relieved** by

ASMETHOD

A	**Age/appearance**
S	**Self** or **someone else**
M	**Medication**
E	**Extra** medicines
T	**Time** persisting
H	**History**
O	**Other** symptoms
D	**Danger** symptoms

WWHAM

W	**Who** is the patient?
W	**What** are the symptoms?
H	**How** long have the symptoms been present?
A	**Action** taken
M	**Medication** being taken

Conclusion

Deciding to prescribe a patient a medicine (or medicines), or deciding to stop an already prescribed medicine, or simply not doing anything for them involving medicines is challenging. Understanding how decisions are made is critical in patient safety. Developing the professional insight and humility which lay bare the limitations humans have when making decisions is crucial. In a busy practice setting, it may seem onerous to have to undertake what may appear to be a very slow and deliberate process to reach a decision. It is true that the mastery of the use of hypothetico-deduction takes time to embed in practice and become second nature. At the most fundamental level, good decisions are usually the ones you can remember making. These have often involved some level of active cognition (system 2 thinking) (Kahneman, 2011). Even for those clinicians whose practice evolves to the point where their level knowledge and expertise allows the use of gestalt, their perceptions of concepts such as proximity and similarity are still tested deductively, and are not unconscious or reactive (system 1 thinking). Patients are treated by human beings because of their ability to provide humanist care. Computers, robots and AI may contribute to improvements in safety in healthcare in the same way they have in aviation, but who would get on a pilotless plane?

Case Study 5.1

Following a pre-alert call from the ambulance service, a 78-year-old female (Mrs G) is brought into the resuscitation room of the Emergency Department with general malaise, dehydration, increased confusion, strong offensive-smelling urine, reduced urine output and pyrexia.

As attending clinician, the Advanced Clinical Practitioner (Advanced Paramedic) listens intently to the handover from the ambulance crew, seeking further clarification on a number of points from all those present. Further collateral history is also sought from the family member present to aid with the ongoing management of the patient.

The family member recalls a three-week history of increased pain and discomfort in the patient's pelvis/suprapubic area, which they thought was related to her osteoarthritis, in particular her chronic hip pain. Mrs G had chosen to self-medicate with over-the-counter ibuprofen and paracetamol for the last 7–10 days, which has had limited effect in managing her discomfort. She has also experienced increased frequency of urination over the last few days, which is dark in colour with decreasing volumes passed. Mrs G has taken a dramatic turn for the worse over the last 24–48 hours and is now confused.

PMH: Chronic Kidney Disease (CKD 3a) [CKD3a is a moderate decrease in eGFR without other evidence of kidney disease], osteoarthritis

DH: paracetamol 1g (QDS), ibuprofen 400mg (OTC/PRN)

Allergies/intolerances: penicillin

SH: lives alone (widowed), regular family visits, non-smoker, denies alcohol, largely self-caring

An initial ABCDE assessment was undertaken:

A = Patent and self-maintained, dry mucosa and lips

B = RR20 shallow, SpO2 95% with four litres of oxygen via a nasal cannula (in situ), bilateral/equal air entry on auscultation, chest clear with no added sounds. No evidence of cough/phlegm/haemoptysis

C = HR 120, BP 88/62, equal radial pulses, pale, not diaphoretic, calf(s) S&NT, no peripheral oedema

D = Rousable, GCS 12/15 (E3 V4 M5), PERL, confused, FAST negative

E = Tenting skin, dehydrated, reduced urine output, BM 4.6 mmol, pyrexia 38.2 °C

Initial working diagnosis: 1. ?Urosepsis and/or 2. ?Dehydration +/- acute kidney injury (AKI)

Immediate resuscitation was commenced in accordance with national sepsis and AKI management guidelines, namely: National Institute of Care and Health Excellence (NICE, 2016) *Sepsis: recognition, diagnosis and early management*, NICE Guideline NG51; Levy, et al (2018) *The Surviving Sepsis Campaign Bundle: 2018 Update*; and National Institute of Care and Health Excellence and UK Renal Registry (2016) *Guidelines for Medicines Optimisation in Patients with Acute Kidney Injury*; local Trust guidelines available online were also used.

Intravenous (IV) access was gained with a number of blood samples taken for analysis – these included: full blood count (FBC), initial profile (IP), including urea & electrolytes (U&Es) and C-reactive protein (CRP).

The following treatment regime was also commenced:

1. Oxygen therapy was continued to maintain SpO2 >94%.

2. Blood cultures were taken (prior to antibiotic use).

3. Fluid challenge was initiated.

4. Lactate was measured using a venous blood gas (VBG).

5. |Urine output was measured following the insertion of a urinary catheter and fluid chart commenced.

6. Antibiotic administration in accordance with local antibiotic guidelines.

7. Sepsis screening was performed: urinalysis and chest x-ray.

Blood results of note:

FBC – Raised white cell count (WCC) 24.2 with neutrophilia of 19.2

Biochem – reduced eGFR 24 (CKD 4) [Her normal eGFR 55 (CKD 3a)] with raised creatinine 136

CRP 98

VBG – pH 7.34 and Lactate 3.0

The FBC results indicate a significantly raised white cell count and neutrophilia suggestive of a severe systemic bacterial infection and increased haematocrit reading suggestive of dehydration.

Mrs G already has reduced renal function with chronic kidney disease (CKD3a). However, the biochemistry results indicate a significantly reduced glomerular filtration rate (eGFR) with raised creatinine levels. This is indicative of an acute kidney injury.

The venous blood gas illustrates a mild acidaemia with raised lactate – again a good indication of severe systemic infection/sepsis in this case.

Prescribing decisions

Given that many medicines are either broken down by the liver and excreted by the kidneys, or directly eliminated by the kidneys, the deterioration in renal function significantly influences the choice of medicines used and must be dictated by evidence-based practice, national and local guidelines.

The decision to stop nephrotoxic drugs must also be taken, and in the management of this case:

1. Stop ibuprofen – given its nephrotoxic effects (Rull, 2016; BNF, 2018c)

Local Trust antibiotic guidelines were used to guide the choice of antibiotic for community acquired urosepsis given the pre-existing chronic kidney disease, new acute kidney injury and penicillin allergy. Local Trust guidelines indicate the use of Ciprofloxacin IV with increased dose intervals (once every 24 hours and not twice daily) if the patient's eGFR falls below 30 mL/minute/1.73 m^2 (BNF, 2018a). Concurrent administration of IV Gentamicin can also be considered, although the dose should again be reduced, with increased repeat dose intervals in severe renal impairment (BNF, 2018b). Gentamicin should be avoided if Mrs G's renal function deteriorates further (creatinine clearance less than 20 mL/minute). For the inexperienced clinician, prescribing in cases of severely reduced renal function and/or renal failure should always be undertaken under the advice of a renal or clinical pharmacist, and the guidance given for many medicines that may potentially be harmful to the kidneys is to either avoid administration, use in reduced doses or use with caution with increased dose intervals. Therefore, the use of prescribing guidelines must be advocated as this serves as a checking mechanism to protect both the patient and the prescriber, reduces the potential for adverse human factors leading to drug errors, and decreases the incidence of harmful drug reactions/interactions.

In the case of Mrs G, one may consider whether the short course of ibuprofen (NSAID) initiated an AKI, which then resulted in reduced urine output and a subsequent UTI? Or did the UTI cause dehydration, which in turn caused an AKI with reduced urine output? This case demonstrates how the treating clinician must remain vigilant to the impact of pre-existing co-morbidities, the potential effects these may have on the pharmacodynamics/pharmacokinetics of any drug administered, polypharmacy drug interactions, and the cumulative toxic effects many medicines exert in cases of poor renal excretion, such as AKI.

Key Points of This Chapter

◆ Decision making is a key part of the role of an independent paramedic prescriber.

◆ Understanding how we make decisions, the variables we consider and the obstacles that may get in our way of making the best decisions will educate the paramedic prescriber to be more cognisant of the complexities of decision making.

◆ Various decision-making theories may help the prescriber to explore and explain their own decision making, with a view to improving practice outcome.

References and Further Reading

Aviation Safety Network. (2018). Air accident statistics. Available at: https://aviation-safety.net/statistics.

Beauchamp, T.L. and Childress, J.F. (2001). *Principles of Biomedical Ethics*, 5th ed. Oxford: Oxford University Press.

Benner, P. (1984). *From Novice to Expert*. Menlo Park, CA: Addison-Wesley.

Benner, P. and Tanner, C. (1987). Clinical judgement: how expert nurses use intuition. *American Journal of Nursing*, 87(1): 23–34.

British National Formulary (2018a). Ciprofloxacin in renal impairment. Available at: https://bnf.nice.org.uk/drug/ciprofloxacin.html#renalImpairment.

British National Formulary (2018b). Gentamicin in renal impairment. Available at: https://bnf.nice.org.uk/drug/ibuprofen.html#renalImpairment.

British National Formulary (2018c). Ibuprofen in renal impairment. Available at: https://bnf.nice.org.uk/drug/ibuprofen.html#renalImpairment.

Carnevali, D.L., Mitchell, P.H., Woods, N.F. and Tanner, C.A. (1984). *Diagnostic Reasoning in Nursing*. Philadelphia: Lippincott.

Charlin, B., Tardif, J. and Boshuizen, H.P.A. (2000). Scripts and medical diagnostic knowledge: theory and applications for clinical reasoning instruction and research. *Academic Medicine*, 75(2): 182–90.

Cioffi, J. (1997). Heuristics, servants to intuition, in clinical decision making. *Journal of Advanced Nursing*, 26: 203–8.

Clinical Human Factors Group. (2018). Website. Available at: https://chfg.org.

Collen, A. (2017). *Decision Making in Paramedic Practice*. Bridgwater: Class Professional Publishing.

Department of Health and Social Care. (2017). NHS becomes first healthcare system in the world to publish numbers of avoidable deaths. Available at: https://www.gov.uk/government/news/nhs-becomes-first-healthcare-system-in-the-world-to-publish-numbers-of-avoidable-deaths.

Dobelli, R. (2014). *The Art of Thinking Clearly*. London: Spectre.

Dowie, J. and Elstein, A. (1988). *Professional Judgement: A reader in clinical decision making*. Cambridge: Cambridge University Press.

Dweck, C.S. (2006). *Mindset: The New Psychology of Success*. New York: Random House.

Elstein, A.S. and Schwarz, A. (2002). Clinical problem solving and diagnostic decision making: selective review of the cognitive literature. *British Medical Journal*, 423(7339): 729–32.

Gallagher, A., Vyvyan, E., Juniper, J., Snook, V., Horsfield, C., Collen, A. and Rutland, S. (2016). Consensus towards understanding and sustaining professionalism in paramedic practice. *British Paramedic Journal*, 1(2): 1–8.

Gambrill, E. (2012). *Critical Thinking in Clinical Practice*, 3rd ed. Hoboken, NY: John Wiley.

Hamers, J.P.H., Huijer Abu Saad, H. and Halfens, R.J.G. (1994). Diagnostic process and decision making in nursing: a literature review. *Journal of Professional Nursing*, 10(3): 154–63.

Hamm, R. (1988). Clinical intuition and clinical analysis: expertise and the cognitive continuum. In J. Dowie and A. Eisten (eds), *Professional Judgement: A reader in clinical decision making*. Cambridge: Cambridge University Press.

Kahneman, D. (2011) *Thinking Fast and Slow*. London: Penguin.

Kant, Immanuel, trans. Jonathan Bennett. (2008). *Grounding for the Metaphysics of Morals*, 3rd ed. Indianapolis: Hackett.

Klein, G.A., Orasanu, J.M. and Calderwood, R. (1993). *Decision Making in Action: Models and methods*. Norwood, NJ: Ablex.

Korn, D. (2016). Barriers to critical thinking. Available at: http://learntoprepare.com/2011/06/barriers-to-critical-thinking.

Levy, M.M., Evans, L.E. and Rhodes, A. (2018). The Surviving Sepsis Campaign Bundle: 2018 update. Available at http://www.survivingsepsis.org/SiteCollectionDocuments/Surviving-Sepsis-Campaign-Hour-1-Bundle-2018.pdf.

Reason J. (2000). Human error: models and management. *British Medical Journal*, 320(7237):768–70.

Robson, D. (2011). A brief history of the brain. *New Scientist*, 2831(2011).

Hamilton, W. (1862). *Discussions on Philosophy and Literature, Education and University Reform*. 3rd ed. Madison, WN: Blackwood, 1866.

McCaffery, M. (1968). *Nursing Practice Theories Related to Cognition, Bodily Pain, and Man–Environment Interactions*. Los Angeles: University of California at Los Angeles Students' Store.

Muir, N. (2004). Clinical decision making: theory and practice. *Nursing Standard*, 18(36): 47–52.

National Institute for Health and Clinical Excellence (NICE) (2018). Website. Available at: https://www.nice.org.uk.

National Institute of Health and Care Excellence (NICE) (2016). Sepsis: recognition, diagnosis and early management. NICE Guideline NG51 (updated September 2017) Available at: https://www.nice.org.uk/guidance/NG51/chapter/Recommendations#managing-and-treating-suspected-sepsis-in-acute-hospital-settings.

National Institute of Health and Care Excellence (NICE) and the UK Renal Registry (UKRR) (2016). Think kidneys – guidelines for medicines optimisation in patients with acute kidney injury. Available at: https://www.thinkkidneys.nhs.uk/aki/wp-content/uploads/sites/2/2016/03/Guidelines-for-Medicines-optimisation-in-patients-with-AKI-final.pdf.

Offredy, M. (1998). The application of decision making concepts by nurse practitioners in primary care. *Journal of Advanced Nursing*, 40: 988–1000.

Rimoldi, H. (1988). Diagnosing the diagnostic process. *Medical Education*, 22(4): 270–78.

Rosenorn-Lanng, D. (2014). *Human Factors in Healthcare*. Oxford: Oxford University Press.

Royal Pharmaceutical Society. (2016). *A Competency Framework for All Prescribers*. Available at: https://www.rpharms.com/Portals/0/RPS%20document%20library/Open%20access/Professional%20standards/Prescribing%20competency%20framework/prescribing-competency-framework.pdf.

Rull, G. (2016). Patient: drug prescribing in renal impairment. Available at: https://patient.info/doctor/drug-prescribing-in-renal-impairment#nav-2.

Syed, M. (2015). *Black Box Thinking: The surprising truth about success*. UK: Hachette.

Thompson, C. and Dowding, D. (2002). *Decision Making and Judgement in Nursing: An introduction*. Philadelphia: Churchill Livingstone.

Tversky, A. and Kahneman, D. (1982). Judgments of and by representativeness. In D. Kahneman, P. Slovic and A. Tversky (eds), *Judgment under Uncertainty: Heuristics and Biases*. Cambridge: Cambridge University Press.

Chapter 6
Prescribing as Part of a Team

Hannah Morris

In This Chapter

- ◆ Introduction
- ◆ Integrated care and healthcare policy
- ◆ Integrated care and prescribing practice
- ◆ Integrated team working
- ◆ Clinical governance
- ◆ Supplementary prescribing and clinical management plans
- ◆ Sharing of information
- ◆ Conclusion
- ◆ Key points of the chapter
- ◆ References

Introduction

This chapter explores how the prescribing practice for paramedics and other non-medical prescribers is facilitated in a team-based approach. It also explores clinical governance for paramedic prescribing. There is a discussion on the use of clinical management plans in supplementary prescribing, and also on how information can be shared effectively across teams for safe and effective prescribing practice.

Integrated Care and Healthcare Policy

Healthcare policy in the UK stipulates the need for services to be collaborative and integrated to ensure safe and effective patient care (NHS England, 2014). Integrated care works to address the needs and demands arising in healthcare from an ageing population and increases in people with multi-morbidity. Evidence suggests that integrated approaches to care provide a more positive experience of patients and families in the navigation of health and social care services (Ham and Walsh, 2013).

Integrated Care and Prescribing Practice

Integrated care not only refers to services working together to achieve the best outcomes for patients, but also refers to healthcare professionals working together to ensure effective team work. Effective team working and the integration of services means that patients receive the 'right care from the right person at the right time' (NHS Providers, 2015). This has meant that in contemporary healthcare practice there has been a development and extension of the roles and responsibilities of healthcare professionals in the development of multi-professional and integrated teams.

In addition, due to fiscal healthcare markets and finite resources in contemporary healthcare, integrated care has meant that professional groups have needed to adopt new roles to maximise their potential in the provision of safe and effective care. Paramedics are a great example of healthcare practitioners who have adopted new roles in new settings and taken on advanced and extended roles, such as independent prescribing, to facilitate timely, safe and effective patient care.

Independent and supplementary prescribing has been a success in contemporary healthcare. It has been able to facilitate timely responses to patient need and a more positive experience of healthcare services for patients and families. This is due to independent prescribers working effectively as part of the wider healthcare team, implementing the principles for effective team working within their prescribing practice.

Integrated Team Working

Working as part of a team is essential in prescribing practice, so it is essential for paramedic prescribers to have an awareness that they are not prescribing in isolation. Although some of the new advanced roles that paramedic prescribers will be undertaking in practice will mean that they are working autonomously, it is important to remember that you are working as part of a team and that you have a plethora of resources to support you in your prescribing practice.

Principles of Integrated Team Working

The principles of team working include (Nancarrow et al., 2013):

- Positive leadership
- Communication
- Personal rewards
- Training and development
- Resources and procedures
- Skill mix
- Supportive team climate
- A shared understanding of roles and objectives
- Quality outcomes.

Leadership

The principles of team working include positive leadership. This may be your responsibility to facilitate within a team, depending on your role. In terms of prescribing practice, you will be a forerunner to paramedic prescribing and will be leading others in the development and evolution of this role. In order to facilitate positive leadership in your prescribing practice, it will be useful to reflect on what has gone well, in addition to what you have found a challenge in your prescribing practice, in order to support others coming into the paramedic prescribing role.

Communication

Communication is a fundamental aspect of prescribing practice. As an advanced level paramedic, you will have developed expertise in communication and interaction processes. In terms of your prescribing practice, the focus needs to be on the interaction you have with patients in gaining a concise and holistic health history on which to base a shared prescribing decision. You will need to ensure excellent documentation skills to evidence the rationale for your prescribing decisions and so that any further decisions can be based safely on what you have done.

Personal Rewards

This refers to the value and satisfaction you will feel from prescribing as part of a team, as opposed to any actual physical reward. This will occur as you make prescribing decisions with your patients and are able to realise the difference you have been able to make as part of a team, in their care. This may be in diagnosing and/or treating of a condition so that the quality of life is improved, or it may be in preventing a hospital admission in the timely intervention of care.

Training and Development

Ongoing professional development as a paramedic independent prescriber is essential. Although once you have your qualification you do not need to update, it is essential that you reflect on your prescribing practice and identify what your ongoing learning needs are. Being part of a wider prescribing team will have its advantages here, as you will be able to learn and share knowledge and experience with other independent prescribers to inform your practice.

Resources and Procedures

These are essential for effective team working in prescribing practice. Policy and procedure guidelines will ensure you have robust mechanisms to protect you as a prescriber and your patients. Resources needed in prescribing practice will inevitably include time, and it is important that as an independent prescriber, you have the time in practice to undertake thorough assessments and to consider your prescribing decisions in an evidence-based approach with your patients. It will be part of your advanced role to advocate for more time to do this in practice if necessary. Effective communication regarding your learning needs and ongoing development within the wider prescribing team should help facilitate this.

Skill Mix

In the wider integrated team in prescribing practice, each professional will have their own field of expertise. It is essential for integrated care and safe and effective prescribing that this is shared. Other professionals will want to access your expertise from your paramedic practice, and you may need their help at other times. Open and honest communication about your skills, knowledge and experience and your scope of prescribing practice will ensure that the patient is treated by the right person and that no undue pressure is placed upon you to prescribe in an area where you do not have the competence to do so.

Supportive Team Climate

By undertaking the principles of integrated team working, a collaborative approach to prescribing practice will be evident. Support is a multi-way concept in prescribing practice and as an independent prescriber, you will find that you will be providing support to other independent and supplementary prescribers as well as seeking it for yourself. It is essential to remember when you start prescribing that it is a new and complex role.

Asking for help when it is needed is crucial – other prescribers have been where you are, and will support any learning and development needs you have. All independent prescribers, from whatever discipline, remember their first encounter with a patient that resulted in prescribing activity, and the nerves, fear and satisfaction that came with this. Integrated care incorporates valuing each other as practitioners; this is particularly true in prescribing practice, and independent and supplementary prescribers will work hard to support each other.

A Shared Understanding of Roles and Objectives

This is essential in prescribing practice. It is imperative that other people understand your role, your prescribing role and your scope of prescribing practice. Likewise, it is essential that you have a clear understanding of the roles of the other professionals you are working with. This allows for clear boundaries and reduces the unrealistic expectations on your practice that can cause conflict.

Quality Outcomes

Undertaking safe and effective evidence-based prescribing practice will support quality outcomes in patient care, and in turn will boost your confidence and competence as a paramedic prescriber and will develop effective integrated team working.

Turn to **Chapter 2** for more on the legal and ethical aspects of prescribing, **Chapter 3** for more detail about consultation and patient-centred approaches to care, **Chapter 5** for theories on decision making and **Chapter 10** for suggestions about undertaking consistent and useful reflective activity, and continuing your professional development·

Clinical Governance

Patient safety is paramount in paramedic prescribing practice; paramedics must prescribe within the law and strive to continually improve their practice to benefit patient care (College of Paramedics, 2018).

Governance structures will be in place if you are employed within NHS and social care organisations, and these must be adhered to as paramedic prescriber. Governance structures for paramedic prescribing practice should include:

♦ clear lines of responsibility and accountability
♦ development of quality improvement structures such as supporting evidence-based practice, audit and access to ongoing training and development
♦ risk management strategies, policies and procedures
♦ poor performance procedures
♦ competency frameworks for prescribing* (College of Paramedics, 2018).

Audit

Audit is an essential part of your prescribing practice. If you are practising as both an independent and supplementary prescriber, each role should be audited separately. Supplementary prescribers should ensure that they meet at least annually with the medical prescriber to review prescribing practice. You should also undertake an audit as a supplementary prescriber to see how many clinical management plans have been followed correctly.

Audit processes should include how many patients you have prescribed for required medical follow up and how many have been successfully treated. It is also good practice to audit the number of patients you decided not to prescribe for or to de-prescribe for, and the outcomes of these prescribing encounters. You can also audit how many times a pharmacist has had to contact you regarding the clarity of a prescription you have issued (College of Paramedics, 2018).

Feedback from patients on your prescribing practice is useful for your reflection and continuing professional development. It is helpful to have feedback from patients for appraisal purposes and to develop your prescribing practice when things have not gone so well, but is also confidence building when positive feedback is received.

---

* The *Competency Framework for All Prescribers* incorporates all competencies required for safe and effective prescribing practice (Royal Pharmaceutical Society, 2016).

Supplementary Prescribing and Clinical Management Plans

Paramedics who hold the independent prescribing qualification and annotation with the Health and Care Professions Council will also be annotated as supplementary prescribers. If you are prescribing as a paramedic supplementary prescriber, you will be prescribing in a team context with a medical prescriber (doctor or dentist).

If you are prescribing as a supplementary prescriber, you must do so within the limits of a clinical management plan (CMP) for an individual patient. A CMP allows you to prescribe certain medicines for certain medical conditions for individual patients in collaboration and partnership with a medical prescriber. CMPs must be written with you, as the supplementary prescriber, and the medical doctor you are collaborating with, and you must have the patient's consent. As a supplementary prescriber, you must never prescribe outside of a CMP. If you are a paramedic independent prescriber and supplementary prescriber, you must adhere to the CMP when prescribing as a supplementary prescriber. This does not stop you from prescribing for this patient for an unrelated condition as an independent prescriber within your scope of practice. If you are prescribing for a certain condition, then this prescribing activity will need to remain within the CMP as a supplementary prescriber (College of Paramedics, 2018); see **Case Study 6.1** for further explanation.

Case Study 6.1

You are prescribing for Mrs Blogs as a paramedic supplementary prescriber under a CMP for her diabetes (as this is a new area to your scope of prescribing practice).

However, during a consultation, you diagnose a urinary tract infection (UTI).

You can treat the UTI as an independent prescriber if prescribing for low-grade infections and antibiotic prescribing is within the scope of your prescribing practice.

The CMP must be recorded before you begin prescribing. This can be a signed paper version or an electronic record. Should the CMP need to be modified, this must be done in partnership with you as the supplementary prescriber and with the medical prescriber; this is also the case should the CMP need to be discontinued in light of any change to the patient status. As the paramedic supplementary prescriber, you have a responsibility to refer back to the medical prescriber with any change in the patient's condition.

Sharing of Information

Prescribing is not an activity that ever happens in isolation. You will be making shared decisions where possible with patients. You must also share the information regarding your prescribing decisions and activity with other practitioners involved in the care who will benefit from the information. You will need to think carefully of the best way to share this information and you will need to consider the General Data Protection Regulation (GDPR) and the Data Protection Act (2018) in the sharing of information.

Ideally, you will have access to contemporary records and to other practitioners' prescribing records, but in practice this is not always the case. IT systems across the NHS rarely 'speak to each other', so it is important that you communicate your prescribing decisions to the appropriate people to ensure the patient's safety and explore all avenues to ensure you have the most up-to-date information on which to base your prescribing decisions.

You must have the patient's consent to share information with other healthcare professionals, and you must explain to them that your prescribing activity cannot be taken in isolation of the wider healthcare team (College of Paramedics, 2018). If the patient refuses to give consent, you should fully explain the risks involved of not communicating your prescribing actions. If the patient continues to refuse, you must consider the best course of action to ensure the patient's safety. This may be to not prescribe. You must document your decision in the patient's notes (College of Paramedics, 2018).

Conclusion

This chapter has highlighted that prescribing practice for paramedics is an integrated approach to care and that prescribing does not happen in isolation. As a paramedic prescriber, you are prescribing as part of a wider healthcare team and should work to ensure that a collaborative approach to care is facilitated with good team working. As a paramedic prescriber, you will need to ensure that clinical governance is maintained to safeguard quality in your prescribing practice.

As a paramedic prescriber, you may wish to undertake supplementary prescribing in collaboration with a medical prescriber, and to do this you must remain within the limits of a clinical management plan and ensure team working with the medical prescriber and the patient.

The sharing of information is essential in prescribing practice in order to ensure patient safety. This needs to occur in a contemporaneous way and with the patient's consent. Data protection should be considered when sharing information.

Key Points of This Chapter

♦ This role you are about to undertake is very important and can be risky. It is vital to access assistance and help as you require it from the multi-professional team and use the support that is available.
♦ Use the CMPs as you have been taught.
♦ Reflect and review your prescribing practice via audit and any other mechanism which will assist you to continue growing in confidence and competence.

References

College of Paramedics (2018). *Practice Guidance for Paramedic Independent and Supplementary Prescribers*. Bridgwater: College of Paramedics.

Ham, C. and N. Walsh. (2013) *Making Integrated Care Happen at Scale and Pace*. London: The King's Fund.

HM Government (2018). *Data Protection Act*. London: The Stationery Office.

Nancarrow, S.A. Booth, A., Ariss, S., Smith, T., Enderby, P. and A. Roots. (2013). Ten principles of good interdisciplinary team work. *Human Resources for Health*, 11(19). Available at: https://www.ncbi.nlm.nih.gov/pmc/articles/PMC3662612/pdf/1478-4491-11-19.pdf

NHS England (2014). *The Five Year Forward View*. London: NHS England.

NHS Providers (2015). *Right Place, Right Time, Better Transfers of Care: A call to action*. London: Association of NHS Providers Foundation Trusts and Trusts.

Royal Pharmaceutical Society (2016). *The Competency Framework for All Prescribers*. London: Royal Pharmaceutical Society.

Chapter 7
Public Health and Prescribing

Hannah Morris

In This Chapter

- Introduction
- Public health
- Public health outcomes framework
- Deprivation and health outcomes
- Public health and the prescribing role
- Antimicrobial resistance
- Antimicrobial stewardship and awareness
- Infection Control
- Conclusion
- Key points of the chapter
- References

This chapter aims to give an overview of the public health aspects of prescribing practice for paramedics. It will outline the importance of incorporating a public health perspective within your prescribing practice in contemporary healthcare settings.

Public Health

Public health is defined as:

> The science and art of preventing disease, prolonging life and promoting health through the organised efforts of society.
> (Acheson, 1988 cited in Courtenay and Griffiths 2010).

Traditionally public health work has been a separate speciality within UK healthcare contexts. Specialist public health roles within health and social care remain. However, with the increase in chronic disease and an ageing population, with longer life expectancy and with finite resources available for health and social care, public health has become the business of every healthcare professional.

Public health work has become common practice and examples are:

♦ monitoring the health status of the population
♦ identifying health needs
♦ building programmes to reduce risk and screen for early signs of disease
♦ preventing/controlling communicable diseases
♦ developing policies to promote health.

Population-Based Public Health Approaches

Traditionally public health had a focus on population health needs rather than individual health needs. Population can be seen as geographical, community, gender, age, disease-related or income-related to define a group of people to be targeted for public health initiatives (Courtenay and Griffiths, 2010).

There has been a steady increase in the number of alcohol-related deaths in the UK since 1994 (Office for National Statistics, 2013). In response to this increase Acheson (1998) suggests organised efforts of UK society in addressing a public health need.

Think about...

What organised efforts could be employed to address excess alcohol use in the UK?

The organised efforts of the UK in a public health approach to addressing excessive alcohol consumption in the UK in an effort to reduce alcohol-related deaths and adverse outcomes and chronic disease include:

♦ NICE guidelines https://.nice.org.drinking)
♦ health services – treatment/advice/prevention strategies
♦ police services – enforcing drink-drive laws
♦ local authorities – running school education programmes
♦ national government – determining licensing laws and tax.

Individual Public Health Approaches

Due to the pressures of contemporary healthcare, with reduced finances available for health and social care, ageing populations with more long-term conditions in addition to a younger population that continues to make poorer lifestyle choices in Western society that will result in increasing health needs, public health policy is now incorporating an individual-based as well as a population-based approach to care. Long-term diseases are closely linked to behavioural risk factors and around 40% of the UK's disability adjusted life years lost can be attributed to obesity, alcohol, smoking and a sedentary lifestyle (NHS England, 2018).

Think about...

What strategies do you employ in your practice that facilitate an individual-based public health approach?

An example of individual approaches to public health can be seen in the 'Making Every Contact Count' (MECC) initiative. MECC is an approach to behaviour change that utilises the interactions that health and social care providers have with people every day to encourage behaviour change that will have a positive impact on the health and wellbeing of individuals, communities and populations (NHS England, 2018). It is possible for paramedic prescribers to adopt a MECC approach within their daily practice during consultations with patients to promote healthier behaviours. This approach can also be adopted for public health-related prescribing practice and this will be discussed later.

The Public Health Outcomes Framework

The Public Health Outcomes Framework (PHOF) is a government initiative that helps public health officials identify trends and areas to target in order to improve health. It sets out a vision for public health in England and the desired outcomes. It identifies target areas for public health practice (Public Health England, 2018). Some of these areas can be adopted in to and considered in paramedic prescribing practice.

Public Health England (2018) identifies current public health areas for targeting in England:

♦ Tackling antibiotic resistance
♦ Reducing incidence of tuberculosis (TB)
♦ Reducing smoking and harmful drinking
♦ Tackling childhood obesity
♦ Applying cutting-edge science to our work
♦ Contribute to improved global health security
♦ Reducing dementia risk
♦ Ensuring every child has the best start
♦ Improving health and wellbeing
♦ Establish prevention programmes (AF (atrial fibrillation), HTN (hypertension), falls etc.)
♦ Reduce the inequality in the uptake of screening
♦ Extend immunisation programmes.

It is possible to identify areas from this list that paramedics can contribute to in their daily prescribing consultations with patients, using the MECC approach to public health. Health promotion and behaviour change through motivational interviewing approaches can address smoking and harmful drinking, as well as improving health and wellbeing.

Turn to **Chapter 8** for further information on motivational interviewing.

Promoting screening programmes and immunisation as part of your prescribing practice is an important part of your public health role. Screening programmes are available for a variety of age groups. Patients should be signposted to the appropriate programmes for their age, as well as the health conditions you are treating that may highlight a risk to their health. For example, a young woman visiting a GP (general practitioner) for the morning after pill should be signposted towards screening programmes for chlamydia. Promoting immunisation is a public health prescriber role. Depending on the scope of your prescribing practice, this could include childhood immunisations or travel vaccinations. A large public health prescribing role in primary care is the flu vaccine programme each year and may inform part of your prescribing role, and this may also extend to the pneumonia vaccine.

As part of your prescribing role, when making prescribing decisions in practice with your patients, it is essential to consider the wider strategic initiatives and interventions you can access as part of your treatment plans to improve health and wellbeing. This can include referrals on to prevention strategies such as falls prevention or pulmonary rehabilitation programmes where they are available. As a paramedic prescriber, you will find that you will develop a wide knowledge of services that would be of benefit to your patients, but may not be available in your local area. As a paramedic and as a prescriber, it is important that you contribute to strategic initiatives in the consideration, planning and commissioning of services that will improve health and wellbeing in a public health approach to care.

Deprivation and Health Outcomes

In **Chapter 3,** we explored the wider determinants of health in relation to health assessment, consultation and prescribing. In looking at Dahlgren and Whitehead's (1991) model to promote equity in health, it can be established that greater deprivation and reduced health literacy can lead to poorer health outcomes. It is of value to reiterate here that as part of your prescribing consultations, it is important to explore any issues regarding deprivation, poverty or lack of health literacy. You are then able to use a public health approach to your prescribing practice, where you can address these by signposting on where appropriate and identifying any areas for health screening in a preventative approach.

Greater deprivation can lead to poorer health outcomes (Buck and Maguire, 2015) where preventative or reactive intervention may be required. These include:

♦ coronary heart disease
♦ smoking
♦ infant mortality

♦ teenage pregnancies
♦ obesity
♦ accidents
♦ substance misuse.

When considering deprivation, poverty and treating people with low incomes, it is important to also consider the psychological impact that this has on individuals as well as treating the physical health problems. In addition, in fiscal markets of healthcare provision and in times of austerity, services and welfare programmes are also cut. This can result in the more vulnerable people in society being adversely affected. Austerity, poverty and deprivation have a huge impact on mental health, which has the potential to cause problems for individuals and communities in the future (McGrath, Griffin and Mundy, 2015). In a holistic approach to prescribing practice, it is essential that paramedics consider the mental health implications within their prescribing decision making with patients.

Public Health and the Prescribing Role

As a paramedic prescriber, you will need to adopt a public health approach to your practice. Contemporary healthcare considerations and public health initiatives 'fit into' the prescribing role in a number of ways. These include:

♦ duty to patients and society
♦ policy regarding the use of antibiotics and vaccines
♦ inappropriate use of medication, including over-use and under-use
♦ inappropriate prescribing, over-prescribing and under-prescribing
♦ access to healthcare provision and medicines.

Think about...

What public health practices will you consider and incorporate into your daily prescribing practice as an independent paramedic prescriber?

Your public health prescribing role as a paramedic independent prescriber could include:

♦ de-prescribing
♦ managing waste
♦ reviewing repeat prescribing
♦ antimicrobial stewardship
♦ managing the misuse of medicines
♦ managing polypharmacy – medicines optimisation
♦ patient health education – MECC
♦ leadership of teams and disseminating knowledge – professional expertise
♦ evidence-based prescribing

♦ cost-effective prescribing
♦ use of and contribution to local formularies.

De-prescribing

De-prescribing is the process of stopping or reducing doses of medicine to manage polypharmacy and improve health outcomes. It requires careful consideration and should be done in a partnership approach with patients, utilising shared decision making. De-prescribing should form a part of your routine consultation with patients as a paramedic prescriber (BNF, 2017).

Questions to consider when thinking about de-prescribing include the following:

♦ Is the drug still needed?
♦ Has the condition changed?
♦ Can the patient continue to benefit?
♦ Has the evidence changed?
♦ Have the guidelines changed (national or local)?
♦ Is the drug being used to treat an iatrogenic issue?
♦ What if any are the ethical issues concerning withholding the medicine?
♦ Would discontinuation cause problems?

Managing Waste

NICE identifies that due to polypharmacy caused by multi-morbidity, the average number of prescription items per person in the UK has risen from 13 to 19 (in 2013). NICE also identifies that adverse events, unplanned hospital admissions and poor outcomes can result from polypharmacy and from people not using their medicines correctly or as prescribed, which contributes to waste. A large amount of money is lost each year from the NHS due to the wasting of medicines. Issues to consider in your prescribing practice that may contribute to the waste of medicines are as follows:

♦ Patients recovering before their dispensed medicines have been taken.
♦ Therapies being stopped or changed because of ineffectiveness or unwanted side-effects.
♦ Patients' conditions progressing so that new medicines are required.
♦ Factors relating to repeat prescribing and dispensing processes, which may cause excessive volumes of medicines to be supplied, independently of any patient action.
♦ Care system failures to support medicines taken by vulnerable individuals living in the community, who cannot independently adhere fully to their prescribed treatment regimes.
♦ Medicines prescribed during a hospital stay being continued unnecessarily when the patient returns home.
♦ Patients stockpiling 'just in case' medicines and reordering repeat medication that they do not need.

It is important to consider the effective use of medicines in your prescribing practice, with a view to any potential unnecessary waste that may be caused as a result of your prescribing decisions. In fiscal healthcare markets, sustainability and the need for cost efficiency is paramount in prescribing practice.

Patient Health Education

The health literacy of patients and the opportunities for health behaviour change using MECC and motivational interviewing strategies have been discussed. This may not be limited to health promotion advice around health behaviour; it may also include informing patients about the best evidence available regarding the choices they may need to make about their health. This could relate to the uptake of immunisation programmes, such as the measles, mumps and rubella (MMR) vaccine for their children. Due to access to the internet, media sources and a plethora of information available, it can be a challenge for patients to reach decisions based on the best available evidence. It must also be remembered that some people, for a variety of reasons, may not have access to the wealth of electronic information and in your consultations, this must be remembered if you are suggesting that your patient should 'find out more'.

Over-use and Misuse of Medicines

Contributing to the waste of medicines in contemporary healthcare is the over-use and misuse of medication. The irrational use of medicines is a major threat to health and leads to a waste of resources. This misuse or overuse of medicines accounts for half the global use of medicines (World Health Organization, 2012). As with non-adherence to medicine regimes, there can be unintentional and intentional over-use/misuse of medicines.

Think about...

Which drugs do you think may be particularly prone to over-use and misuse?

In your prescribing practice, it is valuable to be aware of and consider the medications below, within your practice, as they are prone to be over-used or misused in today's society:

♦ Opioids used to treat pain, such as tramadol, oxycodone and dihydrocodeine.
♦ Sedatives and anti-anxiety medication, including benzodiazepines and the Z drugs (zopiclone, zolpidem and zaleplon).
♦ Stimulants such as methylphenidate used to treat attention deficit hyperactivity disorder (ADHD) and sleep disorders.
♦ Anticonvulsants and mood stabilising drugs such as gabapentin and pregabalin.

Think about...

Which groups of people are particularly at risk of misusing or dependence on POMs or over-the-counter (OTC) medicines?

There are groups of people (see **Box 7.1**) who may present with a greater risk of over-using or misusing medicines, and as a prescriber, you should have an awareness of this within your prescribing practice, as this may influence your prescribing decisions. However, with any prescribing consultation and decision making, this should be person-centred and focused on the individual, their needs and history, and decisions should be reached as part of a shared and collaborative approach.

Box 7.1 – Groups of people who present a higher risk of dependence on OTCs and POMs

- Personal or family history of substance abuse.
- Aged 16–45 years.
- Older people with complex physical and psychological needs further complicated by pain.
- History of pre-adolescent sexual abuse.
- Certain psychological diseases (e.g. ADHD, depression).
- Exposure to peer pressure or an environment where there is drug/substance misuse.
- Easier access to prescription medicines, such as working in health and social care.
- Lack of knowledge and understanding of POMs and OTCs by the prescriber.

It can be a challenge for prescribers to identify where there is an over-use or misuse of medicines. There can be signs and symptoms displayed that may provide cues as to the over-use or misuse of medicines, and as a prescriber, it is important to be able to recognise these and address them with your patients. These include the following:

- Losing medication so that more prescriptions are required – this can become a pattern.
- Seeking prescriptions from various healthcare professionals or practices.
- Requesting a specific drug, as others do not work.
- Stealing or forging prescriptions.
- Appearing intoxicated, sedated or experiencing withdrawal symptoms.
- Mood swings or hostility.
- Increase or decrease in sleep.

If you are unsure in relation to the identification of the over-use or misuse of medicines in your patients within your prescribing practice, seek support from your colleagues in the management of such challenges.

Non-intentional Over-use/Misuse

One of the most common forms of unintentional over-use or misuse of medicines involves paracetamol. Patients may be unaware of the paracetamol content of cough and cold medicines and may take these in addition to paracetamol doses for a prolonged duration, which can have fatal consequences. It is imperative that patients are counselled on the use of paracetamol-containing medicines as part of your prescribing practice.

Over-prescribing

The main cause of concern in contemporary prescribing practice for paramedics with over-prescribing is that of antibiotics.

Antimicrobial Resistance

The term 'antimicrobial' refers not only to antibacterial medicines such as antibiotics but also to antimicrobials, antiprotozoals, antivirals and antifungals medicines (Courtenay and Griffiths, 2010). There has been a developing resistance to antibiotic therapy since 1969. This problem is developing and there is now multi-resistance, with strains of bacteria becoming resistant to two or more unrelated antimicrobials. A high percentage of hospital-acquired infections (HAIs) are caused by highly resistant bacteria such as methicillin-resistant Staphylococcus aureus (MRSA) or multi-drug gram-negative bacteria.

The consequence of such resistance is that it makes infections more difficult to treat, drugs become more expensive in the quest to treat the infections, and the infection remains contagious (Courtenay and Griffiths, 2010). Increased hospital stays are associated with HAIs, which have known adverse effects for patients and results in more costs for already-stretched resources. In addition to financial costs, there is the human cost of increased mortality rate, in particular from MRSA and Clostridium difficile. NHS England (2014) estimates that these 'superbugs' will cause more deaths in the UK than cancer by 2050.

Antimicrobial Stewardship and Awareness

The focus of contemporary health policy in terms of antimicrobial stewardship is focused on antibacterial medicines, such as antibiotics. There is also growing resistance to antifungal drugs and antiviral medication used in the treatment of Human Immunodeficiency Virus (HIV) and influenza (Courtenay and Griffiths, 2010).

In response to the growing concern of antimicrobial resistance, NHS England and Public Health England (2015) have launched collaborative awareness campaigns for health professionals and the public to highlight the problem and promote action. The key messages from NHS England (2015) for prescribers in the effective delivery of antimicrobial stewardship are summarised in **Box 7.2**.

> **Box 7.2 – Key messages for effective delivery of antimicrobial stewardship**
>
> ◆ Right drug, at the right dose at the right time for the right duration.
> ◆ AVOID unnecessary lengthy durations of antibiotic treatment.
> ◆ AVOID inappropriate use of broad spectrum antibiotics.
> ◆ Communication is key – ensure patients have the right information.
> ◆ Consider delayed prescriptions where appropriate.

The considerations listed in **Box 7.2** are essential for paramedic prescribing practice and should be reviewed in every consultation where an antimicrobial prescription is being considered.

Local and national guidelines and formularies will guide you on the correct antimicrobial prescription for the presenting complaint, which will be based on the best available evidence. Each NHS organisation will have an evidence-based guide and formulary for the prescribing of antibacterial medicines due to increased resistance. These will also alert the paramedic prescriber to the correct dose, duration and formulation to treat the presenting complaint. Microbiology can come in useful where there appears to be no improvement in the condition, or formularies offer second-line choices if the patient is unable to use the preferred antimicrobial for any reason, such as allergy or drug interaction. For example, trimethoprim cannot be used with phenytoin (BNF, 2017).

The College of Paramedics (2018) stipulates that paramedic prescribers must always prescribe antimicrobials in line with national guidance (NICE, 2015) and follow local guidelines, based on microbiological advice and best practice guidance.

Patient counselling in the use of antimicrobials is essential in prescribing practice. Not only does this promote adherence, so that the patient will receive the optimal outcomes from their therapy, but education and counselling the patient will ensure the effective use of the medicine. It is hoped that this will prevent further prescriptions being required and will prevent the development of any resistance. It is imperative that patients are educated in the use of antimicrobials, as taking these inappropriately or incorrectly can have potentially serious adverse outcomes. Patients must use the correct dosage and complete the course of antibacterial medicines. Patients should be advised not to share antibiotics or to use other people's antibiotics; this is not appropriate and will increase the risk of resistance and potential side-effects.

When it is appropriate to prescribe antimicrobials as an independent paramedic prescriber, this action should be taken in partnership with your patient. However, when the clinical symptoms are not indicative of a bacterial infection, antibiotics should not be prescribed if they are not indicated. Alternative advice should be given to the patient, or patients should be directed to other healthcare professionals for advice, such as a community pharmacist.

NHS England and Public Health England (2017) have provided a very useful toolkit for prescribers to help focus their practice on antimicrobial stewardship. This is available at: https://assets.publishing.service.gov.uk/government/uploads/system/uploads/attachment_data/file/652262/Antibiotic_Awareness_Key_messages_2017.pdf.

As have the Royal college of General Practitioners (RCGP 2018): http://www.rcgp. org.uk/clinical-and-research/resources/toolkits/target-antibiotic-toolkit.aspx

Under-prescribing

Under-prescribing can have just as much of a negative impact on patient care as over-prescribing. An analysis of primary care records that considered 6% of the population found that one-third of all strokes or transient ischemic attacks (TIAs) occurred in patients where there was a risk of stroke. Prevention medication was indicated, but not prescribed (Turner et al., 2016).

Think about...

What groups of medicines and disease pathologies do you think are most likely to be under-prescribed?

Assessing cardiovascular risk and acting on the outcomes in an evidence-based approach to prescribing practice is essential to prevent adverse outcomes for patients and wider public health considerations. If this is outside of the prescriber's scope of prescribing practice, the patient should be referred on for formal assessment and intervention if there is a perceived risk.

As well as stroke prevention, there is often under-prescribing in relation to osteoporosis, pain control and the use of morphine.

Osteoporosis is increasing in the UK due to the lack of vitamin D absorption as a result of a lack of exposure to sunlight. Under-prescribing in this area may be due to a lack of prescriber awareness and of formal diagnosis. Individual patients should be risk assessed for investigations for formal diagnosis, as not only will this help prevent poor outcomes for patients, it will also save resources in a public health approach in the long term.

Morphine may be under-prescribed due to a lack of confidence in prescribing it in practice and due to the high risk of dependence. The prescribing of opiates should always be undertaken as a multi-disciplinary team approach and decisions made should be based on the individual assessment of each patient.

Infection Control

Effective infection control procedures will reduce the spread of infection and the need for antimicrobials. Good infection control and prudent antimicrobial use by paramedic prescribers will ensure safe and effective care. Infection control procedure should inform everyday practices of paramedic prescribers (College of Paramedics, 2018).

Conclusion

This chapter has discussed concepts of public health in UK healthcare practice. The application of a public health perspective to paramedic prescribing and how this can be implemented in practice has been discussed, using several examples. The importance of antimicrobial stewardship as an independent prescriber has been highlighted in response to public health issues of antimicrobial resistance.

Key Points of This Chapter

- The notion of public health has been explored. How this relates to paramedic prescribers may depend on their place of work.
- Public health interventions, assessment of health risk and health promotion are part of the role of the paramedic prescriber.
- Antimicrobial stewardship is a serious public health issue and the paramedic prescriber needs to be fully aware of the most current advice and where to access relevant 'toolkits'.

References

Academy of Medical Sciences (2016). *Improving the Health of the Public by 2040*. London: Academy of Medical Sciences.

Acheson, E.D. 1988. *Public Health in England: Report of the Committee of Inquiry into the Future Development of the Public Health Function*. London: Department of Health.

British National Formulary (BNF) (2017). *The British National Formulary 74, September 2017–March 2018*. London: BMJ Group.

Buck, D. and Maguire, D. (2015). *Inequalities in Life Expectancy, Changes over Time and Implications for Policy*. London: The King's Fund.

College of Paramedics (2018). *Practice Guidance for Paramedic Independent and Supplementary Prescribers*. Bridgwater: College of Paramedics.

Courtenay, M. and Griffiths, M. (2010). *Independent and Supplementary Prescribing: An essential guide*, 2nd ed. Cambridge: Cambridge University Press.

Dahlgren, G. and Whitehead, M. (1991). *Policies and Strategies to Promote Social Equity in Health*. Stockholm: Institute of Future Studies.

McGrath, L., Griffin, V. and Mundy, E. (2015). *The Psychological Impact of Austerity, A Briefing Paper*. London: Psychologists against Austerity.

National Institute for Health and Clinical Excellence (NICE) (2015). *Antimicrobial Stewardship: Systems and processes for effective antimicrobial medicine use*. London: NICE.

NHS England (2014). *Review on Antimicrobial Resistance*. London: NHS England.

NHS England (2018). *Making Every Contact Count*. Available at: http://www. makingeverycontactcount.

Office for National Statistics (2013). *Alcohol-Related deaths, United Kingdom*. London: Office for National Statistics.

Public Health England. 2017. Antibiotic awareness Key Messages. Available at: https://assets.publishing.service.gov.uk/government/uploads/system/uploads/ attachment_data/file/652262/Antibiotic_Awareness_Key_messages_2017.pdf

Public Health England (2018). Public Health Outcomes Framework. Available at: https://www.fingertips.phe.org.uk/profile/public-health-outcomes-framework.

Royal College of General Practitioners. 2018. TARGET Antibiotic Toolkit. Available at: http://www.rcgp.org.uk/clinical-and-research/resources/toolkits/target-antibiotic- toolkit.aspx

Turner, G.M., Calvert, M., Feltham, M.G., Ryan, R., Fitzmaurice, D. and Marshall, T. (2016). Under-prescribing of prevention drugs and primary prevention of stroke and transient ischaemic attack in the UK general practice: a retrospective analysis. PHOS Medicine. DOI: 10.1371/journal.pmed.1002169.

World Health Organization (2012). *The Pursuit of Responsible Use of Medicines: Sharing and learning from country experiences*. Geneva: World Health Organization.

Chapter 8
Medicines Optimisation

Hannah Morris

In This Chapter

- Introduction
- Long-term conditions
- Medicines use
- Polypharmacy
- Medicines optimisation
- Medicines reconciliation
- Medication review
- Medicines adherence
- Motivational interviewing
- Conclusion
- Key points of this chapter

Introduction

This chapter considers the concept of medicines optimisation for paramedic prescribing practice. It will discuss the importance of medicines optimisation and the closely related concepts of medicines reconciliation and medication review for paramedics, and how this can be incorporated into your prescribing practice.

Long-Term Conditions

A 'long-term condition' is defined as a condition that cannot be cured and that is controlled by medicines and or other treatments and therapies (Snodden, 2010). The prevalence of long-term conditions in the UK has increased, and they are now the most common cause of death and disability in England (NICE, 2015). In 2015, within the UK, 17.5 million people were estimated to have a long-term condition and the number with multiple long-term conditions was estimated at 2.9 million people (NICE 2018). The presence of one or more incurable long-term conditions is termed 'multi-morbidity'.

Medicines Use

Despite medicines being the most common form of intervention to manage and treat ill health in the UK, particularly long-term conditions, the World Health Organization (2003) estimates that 30–50% of medicines used in the treatment of long-term conditions are not used as prescribed. NICE (2015) identifies that the average number of prescription items for any person in England was 19 per year in 2013, an increase from 13 items per person in 2003. The use of multiple medicines is referred to as 'polypharmacy' and with an increase in long-term conditions coupled with an increasingly ageing population, this has become a key issue in prescribing practice for paramedics.

Polypharmacy

Polypharmacy is a term that has been used widely in healthcare practice with mainly negative connotations for some time. Polypharmacy is common in primary and secondary care practice and in care homes, and is a global issue. It is exacerbated by an ageing population and an increase in multi-morbidity and frailty.

Duerden et al. (2013) identified for the King's Fund that polypharmacy is something to avoid in prescribing and healthcare practice, although it can be appropriate at times or problematic at others. They offer dualism in their definition of polypharmacy:

> **Appropriate polypharmacy:** prescribing for an individual for complex or multiple conditions in circumstances where medicines use has been optimised and where the medicines are prescribed according to the best evidence (Duerden et al., 2013).
>
> **Problematic polypharmacy:** the prescribing of multiple medicines inappropriately or where the intended benefits of the medicines are not realised.
>
> This can include issues such as: interactions with other medications taking too many pills, which the patient finds unacceptable (pill burden) taking too many medicines that the patient cannot maintain the prescribed regime medicines being prescribed to treat side-effects (Duerden et al., 2013).

Paramedic prescribers need to know when and how to treat patients appropriately, particularly with ageing and multi-morbidity within their scope of prescribing practice. However, the challenge is in maintaining knowledge of new drugs that come onto the market and being aware of the indications and interactions in patients being treated for a number of conditions, which may often be outside of your scope. Consultations with people who have multi-morbidity need to be longer to ensure that the use of the drugs they use is reviewed effectively, and to support de-prescribing or increases in any medication safely and in collaboration with the patient and the wider healthcare team.

Safety

Safety of medicines use is a key issue when making prescribing decisions. Preventable adverse outcomes can be caused by errors which occur through a lack of knowledge, poor systems and protocols, competency deficits, poor communication and interruptions to the prescribing process. Robust professional and organisational systems can prevent errors in prescribing practice and minimise the risk of adverse outcomes. Adverse outcomes not only affect patient experience and health negatively, but also create a burden for organisations and the NHS as a whole. Transfer between hospital wards, care providers and primary and secondary care results in a greater risk of unintended changes to medicines, as does admission and discharge from hospital. NICE (2015) estimates that when people transfer between care settings, 30–70% of them have an error or unintended change made to their medicines.

Medicines and patient safety is an ongoing issue and there are a number of processes to improve this, such as the MHRA's yellow card scheme. The National Learning and Reporting System, from NHS Improvement (2014), facilitates reflective practice with root cause analysis and learning from experience in organisations where errors occur. NHS England and the MHRA (2014) offer Patient Safety Alerts to minimise harm resulting from medicine error reporting.

The NHS Safety Thermometer (NICE, 2015) aims to measure and support patient safety improvement. This is available across all healthcare settings and allows for identification, measurement and monitoring of contexts of care. The NHS Safety Thermometer is a useful audit tool for organisations as well as individual new paramedic prescribers to audit their prescribing practice over time. This can be useful to identify how your prescribing practice is improving and can aid in the building of confidence in practice.

Patient involvement is essential, where possible, with an individualised approach to prescribing being required. Any prescribing decision you make will not be safe or effective if the medication is not taken as intended. The level of shared decision making by patients in prescribing decisions to aid medicines adherence is also an individual choice that should be respected (NICE, 2009).

Turn to **Chapter 3** for more on patient-centred approaches to prescribing.

Medicines Optimisation

Medicines optimisation is a self-explanatory concept, in that it aims to ensure that medicines are optimised to ensure effective use, and to treat and support the management of long-term conditions and multi-morbidity with the appropriate use of polypharmacy.

Before medicines optimisation, the term 'medicines management' was used in prescribing and healthcare practice. Medicines management was led by pharmacy teams to determine how medicines were used by patients and in the NHS, whereas medicines optimisation reflects and focuses on the actions in medicines use by all health and social care practitioners with patient involvement and collaboration across services (NICE, 2015).

The Royal Pharmaceutical Society (2013) identifies four guiding principles to support the process of medicines optimisation in practice that aim to improve patient outcomes:

♦ aim to understand the patient's experience
♦ evidence-based medicines choice
♦ ensure medicines use is as safe as possible
♦ make medicines optimisation part of routine practice.

These four principles embed patient-centred, evidence-based, safe and effective prescribing practice. Medicines optimisation for paramedic practice is not just about considering the volume and cost of drugs used in your prescribing practice, but also considering how well your patients are supported to use their medicines effectively and safely. This may be through your consultation process and patient counselling, but also referring on to other services, including in the third sector (such as charitable organisations), to support this.

Think about...

What do you need in order to undertake effective medicines optimisation in your prescribing practice?

In order to undertake effective medicines optimisation in prescribing practice, there are a number of factors to consider.

Communication

Clear, concise, effective communication is essential in all aspects of prescribing practice. You will need to be able to effectively relay complex information to patients and elicit their understanding of the prescribed regime in order to ensure safety and efficacy. Effective communication is essential when patients are transferred from one care setting to another.

You will need to document clearly what prescribing decisions have been made and give a rationale. You may also need to identify what options have been rejected and why in order to inform future decision making.

Collaboration

Collaborative practice is a key theme of contemporary healthcare practice. This is essential in prescribing practice to ensure patient safety and wellbeing. Collaboration with colleagues across services, especially when there has been a transfer in care, is paramount to ensure there are no errors in medicine. This can be challenging for new prescribers. If in a transfer of care – for example, on hospital discharge – you identify a prescribing error, it can be difficult as a new prescriber to challenge the prescribing practice of another healthcare professional if you identify anomalies. However, this is essential to do, not only as a professional registrant, but also for patient safety. This can be done in a collegiate and reflective approach to ensure there is learning and an improvement in practice. Likewise, if your prescribing practice is challenged, to have identified your rationale for your decision in the patient's records will help you reflect on why and how you reached the decision you did so that you can reflectively critique this should you be required to do so.

Turn to **Chapter 10** to explore various means of improving your reflective practice.

Sharing of Information

All information regarding the patient and their medicines use must be shared between settings and healthcare professionals, especially when a patient is transferred from one care setting to another. All information needs to be documented. This information should include the following:

- The patient's GP.
- Carer, family and next-of-kin details.
- Details of medicines the patient is taking, including OTC and complementary medicines. This should include name, strength, formulation, dose, timing, frequency and duration. It should also include information on how the medicines are taken and what they are taken for.
- Changes to medicine regimes.
- Date of last dose of medicines that are weekly or monthly.
- What information has been given to the patient and the carer/family regarding medicines and their use.
- Any information on when medicines should be reviewed.

Toolkits to Aid Prescribing

Toolkits are available to assist prescribers in making safe decisions and to effectively manage high-risk medicines in medication reviews. An example of this is the STOPP/START toolkit (NHS Herefordshire CCG, 2016). This provides an evidence-based screening tool for the use of potentially inappropriate prescriptions in older people and a screening tool to alert prescribers to the correct treatments.

The World Health Organization (2003) provides decision-making aids to help facilitate shared decision making with patients that are adaptable for prescribing practice for use by paramedics. These are available online with a range of other aids from other sources within the NHS and social care.

The BNF will be your greatest resource as a prescriber. This may sound obvious due to it being the compendium of all drug-related information; however, it is important to note that there is also other useful information included in the paper copies. There are useful guides on how to use the BNF effectively, general guidance, drug interaction, prescription writing, prescribing in renal and liver disease as well as the emergency supply of medicines. The preliminary chapters and appendices in the BNF will be a great resource for paramedics in their prescribing practice.

Turn to **Chapter 5** to read more about the process of decision making and how to improve your practice.

Discharge Safety

When discharging a patient from your care or receiving an admission into your service, it is essential to maintain safety. Safety can be complemented by sending all the patient's medication information to their community pharmacy or to the hospital pharmacy as appropriate. Ensure that you have the patient's consent to do this with regard to the sharing of personal information.

It is essential that a patient has a full list of their medicines and their indications when being transferred between services, and that any changes to the medication regime are also highlighted on this list.

It is of value to consider some additional support for some people when there has been a transfer of care setting. This could include such support as district or practice nurse input, or pharmacist follow up. This may be particularly relevant for older people, and people of any age with multi-morbidity and polypharmacy.

Turn to **Chapter 2** to review your legal and ethical obligations as a prescriber.

Technical Knowledge of Processes for Managing Medicines

As prescribers, paramedics should be aware of the processes of medicines management, issue and supply within the local area. This should include the general life cycle of the prescription, dispensing and supply of medicines through pharmacy, remuneration and different prescribers' formularies and their scope of prescribing, such as community nurse prescribers, and supplementary and independent prescribers.

Community nurse prescribers are able to prescribe from a limited formulary of mainly dressings, analgesia, emollients, aperients and appliances when they have undertaken the relevant education course.

Independent prescribers are healthcare practitioners who are responsible and accountable for the assessment of diagnosed or undiagnosed conditions and for which decisions about the clinical management are required, including prescribing. Independent prescribers are advised to prescribe generically unless it is not clinically appropriate to do so or if there is no non-branded product available (BNF, 2017).

Supplementary prescribers work in partnership with a medical prescriber (a doctor or a dentist) and can prescribe a limited range of drugs for specifically identified individual patients within a clinical management plan, but only with the patient's permission (BNF, 2017).

Paramedic prescribers will also need to know how their own prescribing practice will be monitored within the employing organisation. This will vary within each organisation, with acute trusts having their own monitoring systems, but in primary care this may well include the use of ePACT data. ePACT data (electronic prescribing analysis and costing) is the data collected by the NHS Business Services Authority based on the prescriptions dispensed by pharmacies. The prescriptions are collated by Clinical Commissioning Groups, GP practices and individual prescribers, and the figures can then be viewed to monitor prescribing trends. This is where your prescribing practice is monitored in terms of your prescribing and this is feedback to you through the medicines management team in your organisation for your reflection and for cost analysis. This process will also help your managers ensure you are prescribing within your scope of prescribing practice and utilising an evidence-based approach. Wider strategic medicines management knowledge will also be required, such as the roles and responsibilities of the pharmacy and medicines management team, and the process of activities undertaken, such as the publishing of local evidence-based formularies.

Therapeutic Knowledge of Medicines Use

Obviously, as a paramedic prescriber, you will be expected to have a therapeutic knowledge of medicines use and their indications. While this knowledge may not be in-depth for every medicine in the BNF, it will be for the medicines you will be prescribing within your scope of prescribing practice. You should be able to demonstrate a good working knowledge of the medicines within the disease areas in which you will be prescribing, even if certain drugs may not be within your scope of prescribing practice. You will be well aware that, as a professional, referring on to a more appropriate healthcare professional when you are outside of your knowledge base and scope of prescribing practice or unsure is paramount for safety and efficacy.

Turn to **Chapters 4** and **9** for more detailed information on pharmacology.

Medicines Reconciliation

Medicines reconciliation forms part of the medicines optimisation process. Medicines reconciliation is the process of identifying an accurate list of a patient's current medications and comparing this with the actual medicines in current use. This will then provide an accurate and contemporaneous list of the medicines that the patient is using. This should also include consideration of any OTC medicines used and any complementary therapies taken. This process should occur whenever there is a change in or transfer of care setting to prevent errors in prescribing practice and to ensure that no adverse outcomes occur in terms of drug interactions. In primary care this should occur at least 24 hours following transfer of care setting or discharge. In secondary care this should occur when there is any transfer within or out of the setting, such as a ward transfer or a transfer to another unit (NICE, 2015).

Medication Review

Medication review is another component of effective medicines optimisation. A medication review is a 'structured, critical examination of a person's medicines with the objective of reaching an agreement with the person about treatment, optimising the impact of their medicines, minimising the number of medication related problems and reducing waste' (NICE, 2015).

This process of medication review is of particular relevance for older people and people of any age with polypharmacy and long-term health problems. Paramedic prescribers undertaking medication review should take into account the patient's views and understanding of their own medicines in a person-centred approach, and any views, concerns or understandings of the family or the carer. There should be a focus on any risk factors for developing any adverse reactions, such as a change in medicine regime, altered blood chemistry or dietary changes. There should be consideration of the safety and effectiveness of how the patient is using their prescribed medication and if this is being used as prescribed and in line with the current evidence base or national guideline for this medicine. Paramedic prescribers should also consider what monitoring and follow-up processes need to be initiated following the medication review to ensure safety and efficacy of use.

 Turn to **Chapter 3** to review history taking and consultation.

Medicines Adherence

Between one-third and a half of all prescribed medicines for long-term conditions are not being taken as recommended, which can result in personal and economic costs (NICE, 2009).

Adherence is now thought to be an outdated and paternalistic term as contemporary healthcare policy now reflects a person-centred and collaborative approach between practitioners and patients. Terms such as 'concordance' reflect a more collaborative partnership approach.

However, in terms of the effective use and management of medicines, adherence is still applied. Adherence presumes an agreement between the prescriber and the patient about the prescriber's recommendations for the use of a medicine (NICE, 2009), and adherence in terms of the degree to which the patient actions that advice. Non-adherence indicates that the patient has not followed the advice, which can result in the misuse of medicines, lack of improvement in health and condition, and limiting the beneficial properties of the medicine being used.

Non-adherence to medication regimes should not be regarded as the fault of the patient. It is reflective of a lack of collaboration and perhaps a failing of the prescriber to reach a shared decision with the patient or to provide full clear and relevant information when making the prescription.

Addressing non-adherence should include consideration of why the medication is not being used as prescribed. Unintentional non-adherence is when the patient would like to follow the prescribed regime but is unable to for extrinsic reasons, such as a lack of understanding, inability to resource the treatment, or memory loss. Intentional non-adherence is when there is a deliberate decision not to follow the treatment for whatever reason, due to beliefs or preference.

While individual care interventions can be initiated to address unintentional non-adherence, other strategies need to be employed to address intentional non-adherence. This can include an open and honest discussion with a non-judgemental approach as to why this is occurring in a patient-centred approach. There can also be a discussion on what ideas and beliefs and barriers prevent adherence, and how these can be overcome. It is important to review this as part of the medicines optimisation and review process, as ideas and beliefs can change over time (NICE, 2009).

Motivational Interviewing

Another strategy for encouraging adherence to medicines is motivational interviewing. Motivational interviewing is beneficial in promoting behaviour change in a range of healthcare settings and this is also applicable to prescribing practice and medicines adherence, where simply giving advice to change can be ineffective.

Rather than the giving of information and advice, motivational interviewing is a process of facilitating a more 'guiding' rather than directive style, eliciting the patient's own motivation to change and by encouraging talk of change. Using this approach, patients are able to identify why and how their behaviour may change, and the practitioner becomes a 'helper' in the change process through expressing acceptance of the patient and their behaviour.

Ambivalence and a lack of understanding can result in a reluctance to alter behaviour in terms of medicines adherence. Ambivalence can be overcome by working with the patient's motivation and values, with the prescribing practitioner working collaboratively, bringing professional paramedic expertise to the relationship. By utilising effective communication that is empathetic, supportive change in behaviour can occur.

For the practical application of motivational interviewing to healthcare, Miller and Rollnick (2008) identify five principles:

♦ Express empathy through reflective listening.
♦ Develop discrepancy between the patient's goals or values and the current behaviour.
♦ Avoid argument and direct confrontation.
♦ Adjust to client resistance rather than opposing it directly.
♦ Support self-efficacy and optimism.

Paramedic prescribers will be well versed in empathy and reflective listening. Using empathy and reflective listening, you will be able to identify what patients say they want or do and what they actually do in response to their health needs. Identifying the difference and explaining this in a supportive context to your patients allows for the opportunity to identify and implement any behaviour change interventions through a motivational interviewing approach. For example, a patient may say that they may want to improve their cardiovascular risk factors and that they are taking a statin, but there is a new prescription of a packet of simvastatin unopened on the side. The identification of such behaviours can be addressed in a supportive non-judgemental context and discussed with patients to explore why this is happening and how they may alter their behaviour in order to elicit change.

The next phase of motivational interviewing is to roll with patient resistance to change or to the interventions in which they are not participating.

By rolling with patient resistance, the practitioner is undertaking reflection and it is through reflection and repeating what the patient has said in a neutral way that allows for the motivational interviewing approach, for example:

Patient: 'I am not taking that pill as it doesn't work.'
Paramedic prescriber: 'You can see no use for that pill at the moment.'

Responding to the patient in this neutral way rather than offering professional advice or a reprimand or giving further direction may elicit an opposite response from the patient. This could be an opportunity for the patient to see where and how this pill might work. For example, the patient may go on to say 'I am not sure how it works', opening up the chance for discussion, or 'it makes me feel sick', which again opens up the discussion.

Another approach of rolling with resistance is the amplified reflection:

Patient: 'I don't know why my daughters worry about me, that pill does nothing for me.'
Paramedic prescriber: 'I can see that your daughters worry unnecessarily about you.'

This type of reflective dialogue gives the patient the opportunity to identify what they could do and why; the patient is likely to discuss in more depth why they feel their daughters worry in relation to the pill in question, opening up a discussion about what they could do to reduce the worry of their children. The practitioner engages with stage 5 of the principles of motivational interviewing when this is identified and encourages any optimism and self-efficacy to elicit change in medicines adherence (Miller and Rollnick, 2008). For example, this could be exploring why the pill is not taken and working with the patient to reach a conclusion on what they can do themselves to improve the situation.

Conclusion

In this chapter we have explored the process and concept of medicines optimisation from the prescribing perspective of paramedic practice. This process is more than making a list of 'current medication' on which to base your prescribing decision. It is a patient-centred approach to collaborative prescribing practice across healthcare services to ensure patient safety and the safe and effective use of medicines in practice. Using motivational interviewing and facilitative approaches, paramedic prescribers can employ medicines optimisation within their practice with a focus on increasing medicines adherence and thereby improve patient outcomes and experience, and managing waste and costs in fiscal NHS markets.

Key Points of This Chapter

♦ Medicines optimisation is key to ensure effective use of medicines, particularly in the management of long term conditions and multimorbidity, due to a higher incidence of polypharmacy. Polypharmacy should be appropriate and therefore paramedic prescribers should ensure adequate time for consultations with patients with multimorbidity.

♦ Safety is paramount in prescribing practice and should be ensured at all times in medicines use, but in particular when patients are transferred from one context of care to another. Paramedic prescribers should reflect on their own prescribing practice and learn from errors and clinical incidences reported through NHS safety systems to enhance good prescribing practice.

♦ Medicines optimisation should be patient centred and any decisions should be made in partnership with patients. This should help improve patient experience and outcomes, improve safety and decisions should always take an evidence-based approach concurrent to the context of care delivery (Royal Pharmaceutical Society 2016). Working collaboratively with other healthcare practitioners and prescribers, with effective communication can help support this process, as can the use of evidence-based toolkits to support prescribing practice.

References

British National Formulary (BNF) (2017). *The British National Formulary 74, September 2017–March 2018*. London: The BMJ Group.

Duerden, M., Avery, T. and Payne, R. (2013). *Polypharmacy and Medicines Optimisation: Making it safe and sound*. London: The King's Fund.

Herefordshire Clinical Commissioning Group (2016). The STOPP/ START Toolkit; Supporting Medication Review. Herefordshire: Herefordshire CCG. Available at: https://www.herefordshireccg.nhs.uk/library/medicines-optimisation/prescribing-guidelines/deprescribing/748-stopp-start-herefordshire-october-2016/file.

Miller, W.R. and Rollnick, S. (2008). *Motivational Interviewing in Healthcare: Helping patients change behaviour*. New York: Guilford Press.

National Institute for Health and Clinical Excellence (NICE) (2009). *Medicines Adherence: Involving patients in decisions about prescribed medicines and supporting adherence*. London: NICE.

National Institute for Health and Clinical Excellence (NICE) (2015). *Medicines Optimisation: The safe and effective use of medicines to enable the best possible outcomes*. London: NICE.

National Institute for Health and Clinical Excellence (NICE) (2018). M*edicines Optimisation, Quality Standard*. London: NICE. Available at: https://www.nice.org.uk/guidance/qs120/resources/medicines-optimisation-pdf-75545351857861.

National Patient Safety Agency (2010). *National Reporting and Learning System.* London: National Patient Safety Agency.

NHS England and MHRA (2014). *Patient Safety Alert: Stage three directive, improving medication error incident reporting and learning.* London: NHS England.

NHS Improvement (2014). *Learning form Patient Safety Incidents.* Available at: https:// improvement.nhs.uk/resources/learning-from-patient-safety-incidents/

Royal Pharmaceutical Society (2013). *Medicines Optimisation: Helping patients make the most of their medicines.* London: RPS.

Snodden, J. (2010). *Case Management for Long-Term Conditions: Principles and practice for nurses.* Chichester: Blackwell Publishing.

World Health Organization (2003). *The World Health Report 2003: Shaping the future.* Geneva: World Health Organization.

Chapter 9
Patient Factors and Prescribing

Jennifer Whibley

In This Chapter

- ♦ Introduction
- ♦ Renal impairment
- ♦ Liver impairment
- ♦ Pregnancy and lactation
- ♦ Paediatrics
- ♦ The elderly
- ♦ Drug interactions
- ♦ Adverse Drug Reactions
- ♦ Individual patient variation: pharmacogenetics
- ♦ Conclusion
- ♦ Key points of this chapter
- ♦ References and further reading
- ♦ Useful websites

Introduction

Chapter 4 looked at the basics of pharmacology and what happens to drugs in the body. However, often in practice, there are variations in terms of how patients handle drugs pharmacologically, so in this chapter we will consider how to apply the principles from **Chapter 4** to different patient groups. Depending on your scope of practice, some of these patient groups will be more or less relevant, but each section will discuss different pharmacological terms and should help consolidate your overall understanding of the subject.

The information here is intended as an overview of each area to give an awareness of the general issues. If you will be prescribing in any of the specific groups discussed in this chapter, then you will need to ensure that you have the adequate level of education and competence before prescribing. This will of course include the practice-based aspect of your independent prescribing course, but references to further reading and resources are included to support your learning.

Turn to **Chapter 2** for the legal and ethical considerations involved in paramedic prescribing.

Renal Impairment

Chapter 4 explained how the elimination of drugs occurs mainly via the kidneys, meaning that renal impairment can have an impact on the pharmacokinetics of many drugs. There are several ways in which renal impairment can cause problems for patients:

♦ Toxicity can occur if renal excretion of a drug or its metabolites is reduced and there is accumulation.
♦ Even if elimination is not impaired, patients with renal impairment may display increased sensitivity to some drugs.
♦ Side-effects of drugs prescribed may cause more problems as they can be poorly tolerated in patients with renal impairment.
♦ Some drugs may actually display a reduced level of efficacy when renal function is impaired

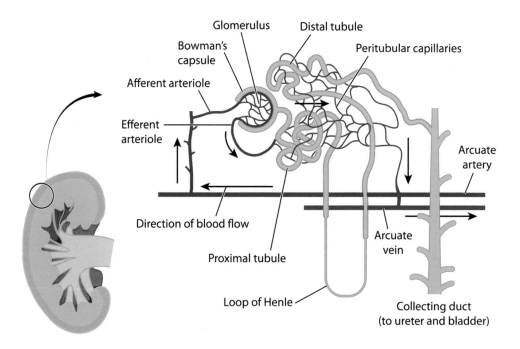

Figure 9.1 – Illustration of the nephrons of the kidney and renal blood supply, which are involved in the filtration and elimination of drugs

Source: © hfsimaging / 123RF.

Figure 9.1 gives a reminder of the basic physiology of the kidney, showing the apparatus involved in glomerular filtration. Drugs that are renally eliminated undergo glomerular filtration and measures that allow an estimation of the rate of filtration are the basis of renal function estimates. There are various such measures that can be used to calculate renal function. How they are calculated varies, but the most common ones use the endogenous marker creatinine, which is a byproduct of the breakdown of muscle. The renal excretion of creatinine happens at a consistent rate and so serum creatinine can be used to assess the rate of renal filtration. An in-depth discussion of these different ways of measuring renal function is beyond the scope of this book, so references to further reading on this subject are included. The main measurement that is reported by laboratories, which you will likely already be familiar with, is the estimated glomerular filtration rate (eGFR). Many sources, such as the BNF, use eGFR when giving recommendations about adjusting drug therapy in renal impairment.

However, it is important to note that as the elimination of creatinine can change in certain circumstances, estimations of renal function are not always reliable indicators.

Factors That Can Affect the Reliability of Renal Function Calculations

♦ Serum creatinine is dependent on muscle mass, so measurements should be interpreted with caution in those who have levels of muscle mass that deviate from the norm, e.g. the elderly, bodybuilders or amputees.
♦ Acute illness that leads to rapid changes in renal function.
♦ Acute kidney injury (AKI).

For a more detailed discussion of estimating renal function, please see the further reading section, for example, the prescribing in renal impairment section in the BNF.

Dosing in Renal Impairment

There are three approaches that can be used to alter dosing regimens to avoid toxicity in drugs where accumulation is a risk. **Box 9.1** provides some examples:

♦ standard dose given at extended intervals
♦ reduced dose given at the usual intervals
♦ a combination of dose reduction and extended interval.

Box 9.1 – Examples of altering dosing regimens to avoid toxicity

♦ Teicoplanin is an antibiotic given parenterally for gram positive infections, such as cellulitis. In renal impairment it is the dose interval of maintenance treatment that is changed rather than the dose itself.
♦ Ramipril is recommended to be started at the lowest dose of 1.25 mg, given once daily as usual. The dose is then titrated according to the response.

Information on the best way to manage changes in dosing can be found from a variety of sources, such as the SPC, the BNF and *The Renal Drug Handbook*.

The Renal Drug Handbook: if you have not come across it before, this book is an invaluable source of information for managing prescribing for patients with renal impairment. It contains monographs for individual drugs, giving detailed pharmacological information and practical advice on dose adjustments (see the References and Further Reading section at the end of the chapter for the full details of this title).

Case Study 9.1

A 72-year-old female patient presents to the GP practice with shoulder pain for the last 2/52.

PMH: type 2 diabetes, mild asthma

Drug history: metformin 500 mg tds, salbutamol 100 mcg MDI 2 puffs prn

You take a history and find that the onset occurred following a period of gardening. You also conduct an examination and conclude there are no red flags and diagnose muscle strain.

What other information would you want to know before prescribing for the patient?

Answer: allergy status. Whether any OTC medicines/herbal remedies are being taken. Also because of the patient's age and the fact they are diabetic and thus prone to renal impairment, when the last U&Es were taken/what they were.

You find after checking the clinical system that the patient has mild renal impairment (eGFR = 55 ml/min). Would this change your prescribing and, if so, how?

Answer: usually simple analgesia such as paracetamol and an NSAID would be prescribed. However NSAIDs can cause AKI and this patient already has renal impairment with an eGFR of 55ml/min. She is also at risk because if she does develop AKI then there is the possibility the metformin she is prescribed could cause lactic acidosis if her eGFR goes below 45 ml/min. There is also the unrelated issue that NSAIDs can cause bronchospasm and this patient is asthmatic. It is only an issue in approx. 10% patients and often patients have taken them OTC without any problem – however, it would need checking.

In this case it is likely that the risk of prescribing outweighs the benefit and prescribing paracetamol alongside non-pharmacological therapy is indicated. Low-dose codeine is a possibility, but we need to be mindful of the risk of falls in the elderly as well as the potential for constipation. It is important to consider any local prescribing guidelines.

Think about...

♦ Always be cautious about prescribing nephrotoxic drugs in patients with pre-existing renal impairment due to the risk of serious consequences.

♦ NICE advises that during intercurrent illness, the risk of acute kidney injury is increased in patients with an eGFR of less than 60 ml/min/1.73 m2. Potentially nephrotoxic or renally excreted drugs may require dose reduction or temporary discontinuation.

♦ Drugs with a narrow therapeutic index require special care in renal impairment – make sure you are familiar with these drugs and, if necessary, get advice when prescribing for a patient on one of these.

♦ Make sure you have thought about where you will look for information and advice when you become a prescriber, e.g. the SPC, the BNF, *The Renal Drug Handbook* and other team members – depending on where you work, this may include more experienced colleagues, pharmacists or even perhaps the renal team.

Liver Impairment

The liver plays an important role in the metabolism and elimination of drugs. As such, liver impairment can alter both drug pharmacokinetics and pharmacodynamics. The clinical impact of these factors is dependent on both the type and the severity of the liver disease. In all patients with severe disease, prescribing should be kept to a minimum.

Some of the possible considerations of prescribing in liver impairment are listed below:

♦ There may be decreased metabolism due to a reduction in or impairment of hepatic enzymes. As the liver reserve is large, it is unlikely that clinically significant changes will be seen unless the impairment is severe. Routine LFTs are not reliable as predictors of which drugs may display impaired metabolism, and there is variation between patients.

♦ Possible changes in distribution may occur with decreased synthesis of plasma proteins can lead to hypoproteinaemia and changes in plasma protein binding. Hypoalbuminaemia can cause an increase in the unbound fraction of highly protein bound drugs, such as phenytoin.

♦ Other changes in the distribution of drugs may occur with water-soluble drugs potentially distributing into oedematous and ascitic fluid. This may cause a reduction in drug concentration at the site of action. This can be exacerbated when drugs that cause fluid retention are prescribed, e.g. NSAIDs.

♦ There may an increase in the bioavailability of drugs that undergo extensive first-pass metabolism.

- ◆ Prodrugs requiring activation in the liver may have a reduced therapeutic effect, though the possibility of reduced excretion leads to the possibility of an unpredictable pharmacological response.
- ◆ Drugs that are excreted via the bile or undergo enterohepatic recirculation via the enterohepatic shunt may shows changes in excretion.
- ◆ Patients may be more sensitive to the pharmacodynamic action of some drugs, e.g. drugs acting on the CNS, the renal effects of NSAIDs and a reduced response to some drugs.

As can be seen from this list, the changes can be complex and multifactorial; as such, it is very hard to make generalisations about prescribing in patients with this condition. The other challenge is the lack of an endogenous marker equivalent to creatinine with which the effect of liver dysfunction on excretion can be quantified.

The BNF features general guidance on prescribing in hepatic impairment as well as information on individual drugs.

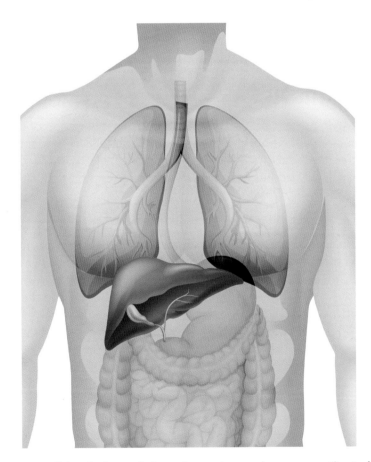

Figure 9.2 – Prescribing in hepatic impairment can change a patients handling of drugs in complex ways

Source: ©blueringmedia / 123RF.

> **Box 9.2 – Example of information on prescribing in hepatic impairment from the BNF**
>
> Warfarin: 'Avoid in severe impairment, especially if prothrombin time is already prolonged.'
>
> See: https://bnf.nice.org.uk/drug/warfarin-sodium.html#hepaticImpairment

A thorough review of the pharmacodynamic and pharmacokinetic implications on prescribing produced by UKMi is available at: https://www.sps.nhs.uk/articles/what-pharmacokinetic-and-pharmacodynamic-factors-need-to-be-considered-when-prescribing-drugs-for-patients-with-liver-disease-2. It is not advocated that you would be making decisions on whether to prescribe at this level of complexity. However, it may be useful to help consolidate your pharmacology knowledge as it a good example of how pharmacological principles can be applied in practice.

Pregnancy and Lactation

There are substantial physiological changes that occur in pregnancy that can alter the pharmacodynamic and pharmacokinetic handling of drugs by pregnant patients. There is also the possibility of the drug having a harmful effect on the foetus, as many drugs cross the placenta. Whilst an understanding of pharmacology can help make the best decisions when prescribing in pregnancy, best practice is not to prescribe at all unless it is essential. A similar approach should be taken in patients who are breastfeeding, as drugs may be transferred to the baby in the breast milk.

Pharmacological Changes in Pregnancy

There are a variety of physiological changes which mean that as pregnancy progresses, variations in absorption, distribution and elimination occur. Some of the main changes are listed below.

Absorption

♦ Gastric and intestinal emptying time is increased by up to 30–40% in the second and third trimesters. This could lead to delayed absorption for some drugs.
♦ Decreased gastric acid secretion leads to a change in gastric pH, which can affect the absorption of some drugs.
♦ Nausea and vomiting can lead to decreased absorption of drugs prescribed orally.

Distribution

♦ The Vd of drugs can change as the volume of plasma increases by up to 50% over the course of a pregnancy.

- The foetus can be viewed as another body 'compartment', which adds an extra level of complexity to how drugs distribute.
- As plasma protein production does not increase in line with the increase in plasma volume, there can be a dilutional hypoalbuminaemia.

Elimination

- Increased renal blood flow leads to an increase in the rate of glomerular filtration during pregnancy.
- Changes in hepatic metabolism can occur, but are difficult to quantify.

The Impact of Prescribing on the Foetus

Drugs can have an impact on the foetus at any time during pregnancy. However, because of the developmental stages that occur throughout pregnancy the risks can differ depending on the trimester. For further information see the references at the end of the chapter, particularly the BNF which contains a section on prescribing in pregnancy.

First trimester

Generally, the first trimester poses the highest risk and prescribing should be avoided unless absolutely essential during this time. This is because the foetus undergoes significant cell division during this time and drugs used during this stage can lead to congenital malformations.

Second and third trimesters

There is a risk that drugs may affect the growth and functional development of the foetus and may cause toxicity in foetal tissues. There is also the risk of neonatal withdrawal if prescribing continues up to birth, for example, with opiates prescribed for addiction or pain.

One of the challenges in this area is the lack of clinical data because of the ethics of conducting clinical trials in pregnant patients. A lot of drug use, as in paediatrics, is therefore unlicensed in this group of patients. There are resources available and advice should always be sought in cases where there is any uncertainty on whether it is safe to prescribe. It also important to ask the patient about whether they are taking any Over the Counter (OTC) medicines or herbal remedies in both pregnancy and breast feeding as these can also affect the foetus or neonate.

Lactation

There are established benefits of breastfeeding and this is encouraged if at all possible. For patients who are prescribed medicines, there is a risk that the maternal dose can partition into the breast milk and be transferred to the child. The clinical significance of this is not always easy to assess, but possible risks must always be considered.

There is information included in the BNF on prescribing in lactation, and drug monographs often include advice on safety. It should be noted that because there is not sufficient evidence to provide guidance, this advice is not always included. The absence of advice does not imply safety. If there is no advice readily available, then more specialist advice should be sought.

Some drugs that can have a pharmacological effect on breastfed infants:

♦ Some sedatives and hypnotics can produce a response, for example, diazepam. This drug poses a particular risk because its long-half life can lead to accumulation.
♦ It is recommended that codeine is avoided in lactation. Although the amount will often be too small to be harmful, there is sufficient inter-patient variation in terms of how codeine is metabolised. This can lead to higher than normal maternal levels in some patients that will produce toxicity in breastfed infants.

There are strategies that can help minimise the transfer of drugs into breast milk and where prescribing is indicated, these should be used:

♦ The maternal dose should be taken after feeding to allow the maximum amount of drug to be cleared before the next feed.
♦ Breast milk can be expressed at a time when the maternal serum concentrations are likely to be at their lowest.
♦ Remember that the selection of drug matters because of its half-life. The shorter the half-life, the more likely it is to clear before the next feed is due and drugs within the same class can have different half-lives.
♦ Prescribe drugs at the lowest effective dose.

Think about...

♦ If a patient is pregnant, even if there is pharmacological management available, always consider if there are non-pharmacological options that can be tried first?
♦ If they do need treatment, make sure it is for the shortest possible time and that a regular review is in place.
♦ Consider the trimester and any risks associated with the pregnancy.
♦ If you are unsure, always get advice.
♦ Check individual drug safety and follow best practice guidance on prescribing in breastfeeding.

Paediatrics

Perhaps the most important thing to remember about the pharmacology of drugs in paediatrics is that this group are not just small adults; they represent a heterogenous group who are constantly changing in terms of their pharmacological response to medicines. The changes in body size, surface area and metabolic pathways mean that it is not just a case of merely reducing the paediatric dose to a proportion of the adult dose.

As children grow and develop, there is a continuum of changes that they go through. These affect the dose that is needed, the efficacy of response that may be seen and the chances of there being an ADR to the drug.

Changes that influence the pharmacological handling of drugs during paediatric development include:

♦ body composition
♦ organ function
♦ drug metabolising enzymes
♦ renal function.

Pharmacodynamics

There is very little data associated with altered pharmacodynamic changes. Most clinical practice is therefore based on observation and experience.

Pharmacokinetics

Absorption

As explained in **Chapter 4**, the absorption of a drug depends on the route of administration used. The rate and the extent of oral absorption depend on several factors, including gastrointestinal (GI) pH, GI transit time and GI contents. Because of differences in gastric emptying and intraluminal pH, absorption can differ in the paediatric population compared to the adult population. Topical agents may also be absorbed differently into the systemic circulation due to differences in body surface area and developmental variation in the composition of the skin.

Some factors that can affect absorption in paediatric patients are as follows:

♦ Gastric emptying and peristalsis is delayed and unpredictable in neonates, with adult values not seen until about six months.
♦ In the neonatal and infant period gastric pH is relatively high, and only falls to adult levels at around two to three years of age. This is due to reduced gastric acid secretion in the early phase of life. What this means is that there is a greater absorption of weakly alkaline drugs through the gut mucosa in infants, whereas weakly acidic drugs are less well absorbed. The altered pH can also have an effect on the degree of degradation of acid-labile drugs. Penicillins, for example, are acid-

labile and so in infants, where the pH is raised, they are less readily degraded, leading to a greater proportion available to be absorbed.

♦ Absorption of fat-soluble drugs can be affected by a decreased level of bile production in neonates.

♦ There is a larger body surface area relative to weight in neonates and infants, meaning that systemic absorption of topical agents may be increased.

♦ The skin can also present less of a barrier to drug used topically in children because the stratum corneum is thinner and the skin has a greater level of hydration.

Routes of Administration

It is important to remember that the route of administration depends on a whole host of factors, including age, disease condition, parental perspective and any issues identified around adherence.

Think about...

When you prescribe how the child is going to take the medicine?

♦ If dosing is based on weight, then consider rounding up or down to make it practical to administer.

♦ Always check with the parents/carer which formulation would suit the child. Sometimes liquids are prescribed automatically when in fact the child finds tablets/capsules easier.

♦ Consider the excipients in the formulation as some can cause problems for children (for example, some liquids contain ethanol, which would not cause problems in an adult, but could in a neonate).

♦ Make sure your directions are clear in terms of both the dose and the volume to be given.

♦ Make sure you have access to paediatric-specific information to support you.

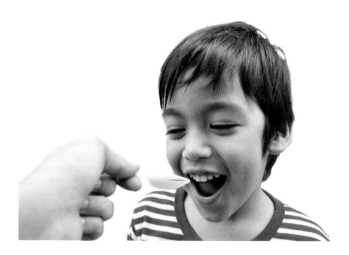

Figure 9.3 – When prescribing, it is important to think about how the dose prescribed is going to be administered to the child.

Table 9.1 – The advantages and disadvantages of different routes of administration in paediatric patients

Enteral Routes		
	Oral	**Sublingual/buccal**	**Rectal**
Description	Drugs in the form of syrup, tablets or capsule are placed in the mouth and swallows. Administration of drugs through the nasogastric or gastrostomy route works in the same way as the oral route.	Drugs placed under tongue/buccal cavity and absorbed in the mouth.	Drugs administered as suppository are readily absorbed in the blood-rich thin rectal wall (e.g. paracetamol diclofenac, glycerine, paraidehyde).
Advantages	Convenient; can be administered by the child or caregiver; pain-free, inexpensive; prolonged absorption in the gut.	Rapidly absorbed; avoids first-pass metabolism in liver; can be administered by caregivers at home, e.g. buccal midazolam as rescue medication in children with epilepsy.	Quick absorption; can be given in children with nausea/vomiting/swallowing problems. Can be used in emergencies at home, e.g. rectal diazepam.
Disadvantages	Compliance can be in issue with some children; cannot be used in emergencies; not sutable for children who are vomiting; undergoes first-pass mechanism in liver so drug levels may vary.	Compliance can be an issue with some children; small doses required hence needs parental/child's understanding and training.	Rectal irritation, so children may dislike it; cultural acceptance; cannot be used in children who have diarrhoea.

Source: Paul, S.P, Whibley, J. John, S. (2013). Challenges in paediatric prescribing, *Nurse Prescribing* (9)5. Reproduced with permission.

Parenteral routes			
Intravenous	**Intramuscular**	**Subcutaneous**	**Inhalation**
One of the commonest routes in paediatric practice. Drugs and fluids can be directly administered in the vein through an intravenous cannula, percutaneous peripheral long line.	Drugs administered in the muscles such as the deltoid and absorbed in the blood steadlily from the muscle, e.g. vaccinations.	Drugs administered in the subcutaneous layer and absorbed in the blood (e.g. insulin in Type I diabetes).	Drugs administered as aerosols and absorbed in the blood (e.g. inhalers, nebulisers).
Immediate onset of action; absorption phase bypassed so useful in emergencies/ sick children; large volume of drugs or fluids, e.g. total parenteral nutrition in premature babies, better compliance if palatability is an issue, e.g. antibiotics.	Rapid basorption achieved in emergencies, such as adrenaline in anaphylaxis; parents can be trained to do it at home; short-term alternative route where intravenous access is difficult.	Can be administered at home with training; bypasses first-pass metabolism in the liver.	No need for injections so painless; rapid onset of action; targeted drug delivery.
Needs skilful insertion of the device by a trained health professional; pain at the site of injection; high concentrations achieved rapidly so dosage calculation needs to be accurate; risk of embolism; children may dislike the sensation.	Pain at the site of injection so children may dislike it; incorrect administration may cause haemmatoma or abcess; trained staff required.	Compliance may be an issue as injection site can be painful; lipohypertrophy at injection sites; repeated use of such sites may lead to dcreased drug absorption. thus to poor control (Wallymahmed, 2004).	Compliance isses as children may dislike the mask or noise; local or systemic effects from swallowing, especially in younger children.

Distribution

As discussed in **Chapter 4**, drugs partition into different parts of the body depending on the composition of the fluid and tissue, as well as the physicochemical properties of the drug. As changes in age lead to changes in the composition of the body, the distribution patterns of drugs can differ depending on the age of the patient.

At birth, the body has a higher proportion of total body water, which decreases with age. Conversely, the proportion of body fat increases in the first year after birth and then decreases gradually before reaching adult levels. These changes can affect the Vd of drugs depending on their tendency to partition into lipid or aqueous environments.

Another variation seen in neonates and infants is that they have a reduced level of total plasma proteins. Drugs that are extensively protein-bound will therefore have a high proportion of unbound drug in the systemic circulation.

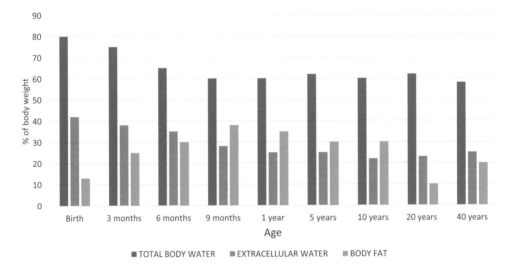

Figure 9.4 – Developmental changes in body composition that can affect drug distribution

Source: Based on data from Gregory L. Kearns, Susan M. Abdel-Rahman, Sarah W. Alander, M.D., Douglas L. Blowey, J. Steven Leeder and Ralph E. Kauffman. Developmental Pharmacology — Drug Disposition, Action, and Therapy in Infants and Children. *The New England Journal of Medicine*. 2003; 349:1157–1167: Available from: https://www.nejm.org/doi/full/10.1056/NEJMra035092.

Metabolism

At birth, metabolic pathways are either absent or incompletely developed, particularly in premature babies. As development progresses, the metabolism of drugs can vary as these pathways mature at different rates. As discussed in **Chapter 4**, the CYP450 group of enzymes are important in drug metabolism. Within this group there are various subsets of enzymes, known as isoforms, that are responsible for metabolising different drugs. **Figure 9.5** illustrates how with age, the metabolic capacity of various enzyme isoforms changes.

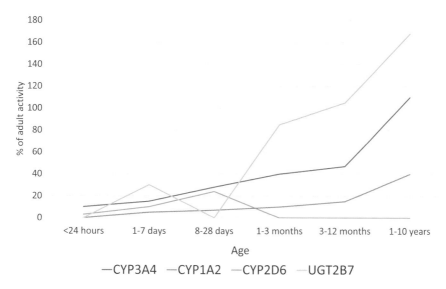

Figure 9.5 – Showing changes in metabolic capacity from birth to ten years of age

Source: Based on data from Gregory L. Kearns, Susan M. Abdel-Rahman, Sarah W. Alander, M.D., Douglas L. Blowey, J. Steven Leeder and Ralph E. Kauffman. Developmental Pharmacology — Drug Disposition, Action, and Therapy in Infants and Children. *The New England Journal of Medicine.* 2003; 349:1157–1167: Available from: https://www.nejm.org/doi/full/10.1056/NEJMra035092.

The reduced metabolic capacity of some systems can lead to the half-life ($T_{1/2}$) of a drug being greater in a child. For example, phenobarbital has a half-life of 70–200 hours in the first few days of life, but by 2–3 weeks of age this has fallen to 20–50 hours.

Whilst it may be unexpected, some drugs actually have a higher degree of clearance in children than they do in adults because of enhanced metabolism. For these drugs, larger doses per kilogram are needed relative to adult doses. One example of this is theophylline, which is used in respiratory disorders. Larger doses per kilogram are needed in children aged 1–9 possibly because of the relatively larger size of the liver in this age group.

Elimination

The process of renal elimination is complex in the paediatric population. At birth, the glomerular filtration rate is significantly less than the rate in infants, older children and adults. If the rate is calculated taking into account body surface area, newborn glomerular filtration is only 30–40% of adult values.

This we may expect given the immature state of the kidneys at birth. What may not be expected is that by the age of 6–12 months, glomerular filtration is equivalent to adult values when adjusted for body surface area and then goes on to actually exceed adult values. This means that the renal clearance of drugs can be greater than in adults for some drugs, which means that sometimes larger doses per kilogram are needed.

ADRs in Paediatrics

ADRs will be covered in a later section, but it is worth noting in this section that paediatric patients are particularly susceptible to ADRs. Make sure you know how to identify and manage an ADR. Also make sure you know how to report an ADR – for more on this, see below.

The Elderly

Changes in physiology are not restricted to the young and throughout life, the human body continues to demonstrate complex changes that can impact on the pharmacological handling of medicines. It is important to understand that ageing is not uniform or consistent. It represents the sum of a variety of changes that occur at different rates in different individuals. It involves functional decline as well as a variety of anatomical and physiological changes, all of which can lead to changes in the pharmacological response of an individual.

An important factor in the older population is the increased propensity for co-morbidities and polypharmacy. This is in addition to the changes that happen as a natural part of ageing. **Figure 9.6** illustrates that functional decline generally begins in the forties and continues in a roughly linear trajectory into old age. It is important to remember that functional change is very variable and the data presented in **Figure 9.6** represents mean figures. **Table 9.2** shows some of the physiological and anatomical changes that can also occur, which affect the pharmacokinetic handling of drugs.

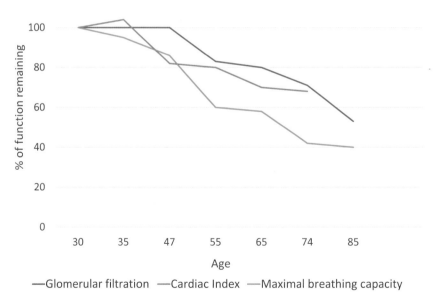

Figure 9.6 – Showing the effect of age on some physiological functions

Source: Based on data from Katzung, B., Masters, S., Trevor, A. (eds) (2012) *Basic and Clinical Pharmacology.* MacGraw-Hill, p. 1052.

Table 9.2 – Showing some age-related changes in pharmacokinetics

Variable	Young adults (20–30 years)	Older adults (60–80 years)
Body water (% of body weight)	61	53
Lean body mass (% of body weight)	19	12
Body fat (% of body weight)	26–33 (women) 18–20 (men)	38–45 (women) 36–38 (men)
Serum albumin (g/dL)	4.7	3.8
Kidney weight (% of young adult)	(100)	80
Hepatic blood flow (1% of young adult)	(100)	55–60

Source: Katzung, B., Masters, S., Trevor, A. (eds) (2012) *Basic and Clinical Pharmacology.* MacGraw-Hill, p. 1052.

Pharmacodynamic Changes

Elderly patients appear to show increased sensitivity to the pharmacodynamic effects of certain drugs. It may be that these changes are actually linked to pharmacokinetic processes that have not been elucidated, but clinical studies certainly indicate that the elderly are more sensitive to many commonly used drugs.

Examples of drugs that elderly patients display increased sensitivity to include:

♦ benzodiazepines
♦ antipsychotics
♦ antiparkinsonian drugs
♦ NSAIDs
♦ antihypertensives.

Pharmacokinetic Changes

As **Table 9.2** shows, there are various changes that happen with age that can affect pharmacokinetic handling. Overall percentage body water decreases, as does lean body mass, whilst percentage body fat increases. This can affect the distribution of medicines.

However, the most important change is the potential for reduced renal elimination, which can lead to prolongation of a drug's half-life and accumulation of a drug in the body. It should be noted that eGFR has limited value in elderly patients and another measurement known as Creatinine Clearance (CrCl) is recommended in patients over 75 years of age. This is calculated using the Cockcroft and Gault formula.

The Cockcroft and Gault formula:

$$\text{Creatinine Clearance (ml/min)} = \frac{(140 - \text{age}) \times \text{weight} \times \text{constant}}{\text{Serum Creatinine}}$$

- Age is in years.
- Weight is in kilograms. Ideal body weight should be used where body fat is likely to be the main contributor to body mass.
- Constant is dependent on gender and = 1.23 for men and 1.04 for women.
- Serum creatinine is in micromol/litre.

Make sure you use the right figure as eGFR and CrCl are not interchangeable.

Key Considerations When Prescribing to the Elderly

- Make sure when prescribing that you have the competence to know how the drugs you are prescribing affect elderly patients. The BNF suggests prescribers limit the range of medicines they prescribe in the elderly to ones that they are thoroughly familiar with.
- Consider whether pharmacological management is needed – is there a non-pharmacological option that would be appropriate, e.g. diuretics used chronically are over-prescribed. They should not be prescribed for gravitational oedema for more than a few days. Instead, increased movement, elevation and support stockings should normally be used.
- Make sure appropriate follow-up and review is in place. Medicines should be monitored and reviewed regularly. Any medicines no longer deemed appropriate should be de-prescribed.
- Consider using a tool to help support in reviewing and stopping medicines, e.g. the STOPP/START tool.
- Consider the risk-benefit ratio when prescribing; this may change in elderly patients.
- Consider the patient as a whole, including co-morbidities, all medication currently taken and the degree of age-related change in that patient.

For further support on this topic, see the references given at the end of the chapter.

The section in the BNF on prescribing for the elderly contains a useful summary that is easy to refer to and includes more detail on the different measurements of renal function.

Drug Interactions

Drug interactions happen when the effect of a drug is changed by the presence of another drug, a chemical or even a food. Because patients are often prescribed multiple medicines it important to be aware of the possibility of interactions an know how to manage them.

Pharmacodynamic Interaction

These interactions occur when drugs have either similar or antagonistic pharmacological effects. If, for example, two drugs are given that both cause sedation, then this can have an additive effect.

Clinical Examples of This Type of Drug Interaction

◆ Diazepam and mirtazapine – both have CNS depressive effects, which can have an additive effect producing CNS effects such as increased drowsiness.
◆ Citalopram and carbamazeprine – both can lead to reduced sodium levels and so when used together, there is an increased risk of hyponatremia.
◆ Warfarin and aspirin – this interaction increases the risk of bleeds due to an additive effect of anticoagulant and antiplatelet action of the drugs.

This type of interaction is normally predictable based on the known pharmacology of the drug.

Pharmacokinetic Interaction

These interactions occur when one drug alters the absorption, distribution, metabolism or elimination of another drug. Because of the complex nature of pharmacokinetic effects, it may not always be possible to easily predict these interactions. Common examples of this kind of interaction may be interactions caused by the induction or inhibition CYP450 enzyme systems that was discussed in **Chapter 4**.

Clinical Examples of This Type of Drug Interaction

◆ Bisphosphates and calcium supplements: calcium is predicted to reduce absorption of bisphosphates and a gap is recommended between ingestion of the different drugs.
◆ Simvastatin and grapefruit juice: grapefruit juice increases levels of simvastatin due to changes in metabolic enzymes, leading to the possibility of severe side-effects, including rhabdomyolysis.
◆ Doxycycline and iron supplements: iron should be taken 2–3 hours after tetracycline antibiotics such as doxycycline as it decreases the absorption of these antibiotics.

When you are faced with the possibility of having to prescribe two interacting drugs, it is important to consider the options, including the risk-benefit ratio of prescribing. Some factors to consider when there is the possibility of drug interactions are as follows:

◆ What information is there on how common the interaction is?
◆ How severe are the consequences of the interaction if it occurs?
◆ Is the interaction dose-related and can the risk be minimised by a dose reduction?
◆ Are there other drugs that do not interact that could achieve the same therapeutic outcome?
◆ If a short course of treatment is needed, can an interacting drug be temporarily stopped?
◆ Is there any monitoring that can be done to monitor for the development of an interaction?

Case Study 9.2

A 66-year-old patient attends an appointment following a one-week history of purulent cough.

PMH: hypercholesteremia, hypertension

Drug history: amlodipine 10 mg od, simvastatin 20 mg on

Allergies: penicillin

Following a full history and physical examination, you diagnose that he has a low-severity community acquired pneumonia.

Question: Based on the NICE guidelines for diagnosing and managing pneumonia, what treatment will you recommend?

Answer: Ideally treatment should be with a penicillin, such as amoxicillin, for five days. In penicillin-allergic patients, a macrolide should be used. Local guidelines usually recommend clarithromycin and this is the drug that would normally be used.

Question: Based on this, would you need to make any adjustment to the patient's other drugs? If so, what would they be and what is the reason for this?

Answer: The simvastatin treatment would need to be ceased for the duration of and approximately one week after treatment with the macrolide to ensure elimination of the clarithromycin. This is possible because simvastatin is for chronic prevention and stopping it for a short time does not pose a risk to patients. This is in contrast to the potentially serious consequences of the interaction.

Adverse Drug Reactions (ADRs)

The World Health Organization's definition of an ADR is a noxious, unintended or undesired effect of a drug when used at therapeutic doses. This does not include toxic reactions, which are produced by above-therapeutic doses.

The definition was written in 1972 by the World Health Organization in a report produced in response to the growing problem of ADRs. Unfortunately, even with increased safety monitoring of drugs, ADRs continue to be of huge significance in practice. **Box 9.3** gives an idea of the burden of ADRs to both patients and the NHS. As a prescriber, it is your responsibility to try where possible to identify patients who may be at risk of an ADR and also to correctly manage patients who present with an ADR. As we will see, this is not always an easy task and so taking time to familiarise yourself with this topic is important.

> **Box 9.3 – Summary of key findings from a study investigating the burden of ADRs on patients and the NHS**
>
> ◆ ADRs account for 1 in 16 hospital admissions and 4% of NHS bed capacity.
> ◆ 70% of ADRs were considered to be avoidable.
> ◆ Many ADRs were predictable based on the pharmacology of the drugs involved and were therefore likely to be preventable.
> ◆ 1 in 6 ADRs was due to drug interactions.
> ◆ Admissions caused by ADRs led to mortality in 2% of patients.
> ◆ ADRs may be the cause of death in 0.15% of all patients admitted to hospital (this figure is consistent with data from the US).
>
> *Source*: Pirmohamed, M. et al. (2004). Adverse drug reactions as cause of admission to hospital: prospective analysis of 18,820 patients. *BMJ*, 329: 15–19.

What this information in **Box 9.3** shows is the frequency of ADRs, the potential severity, but also that many ADRs were in fact preventable based on knowledge of their pharmacology.

Classifying ADRs

The ABCDE classification has traditionally been used for ADRs. The most common are Type A & B, but it is important to be aware of the other types.

Type A (augmented): these are pharmacologically predictable and dose-dependent. As such, they are common and can be managed by dose reduction. They tend to have a low mortality.

Example: postural hypotension on initiation of ACE inhibitors. This is why low doses are used initially and titrated up.

Type B (bizarre): these are not pharmacologically predictable or dose-dependent. They are uncommon and tend to have a higher incidence of mortality. Discontinuation of the drug is necessary. The causes of these reactions may have an immunological or genetic basis.

Example: blood dyscrasias in patients prescribed the antipsychotic clozapine. Patients prescribed this drug are rigorously monitored to identify if they may be developing this ADR. It is still used because it is effective in patients with extremely hard-to-manage conditions who have not responded to other antipsychotics.

Type C (chronic): mostly associated with chronic use leading to some kind of toxic response.

Example: suppression of the hypothalamus-pituitary gland-adrenal cortex by long-term systemic glucocorticoid treatment.

Type D (delayed): the time course of developing these kinds of reaction is not necessarily immediate. Reactions can be seen after treatment has ceased.

Example: drugs prescribed in pregnancy that may cause teratogenesis where the ADR may only become evident after birth. Another example is anticancer drugs that can in fact cause mutagenesis/carcinogenesis and may in fact increase the risk of a secondary malignancy following treatment.

Type E (end of treatment): these reactions occur when treatment is stopped, so include withdrawal reactions and rebound reactions when physiological systems have adapted to the presence of the drug.

Examples: abruptly ceasing opiates after long-term use can cause withdrawal reactions. Stopping beta-blockers suddenly can cause rebound tachycardia due to upregulation of receptors.

Practical Steps to Minimise ADRs

♦ Make sure you are able to apply knowledge of the pharmacodynamic and pharmacokinetic properties of any drugs you are initiating to your patient.
♦ Make sure you look carefully at the patient's drug history to look for the potential for any drug interactions that may lead to an ADR, e.g. NSAIDs and SSRIs leading to an increased risk of GI bleed.
♦ Make sure you ask about any OTC and herbal products as these can influences the risk of an ADR
♦ Consider the patient's medical history and the possibility of an ADR, e.g. starting drugs that cause postural hypotension in a patient at risk of falls.
♦ Utilise any prescribing support available to you, such as computerised alerts on prescribing systems.
♦ If there is a risk of an ADR, consider other options, e.g. non-pharmacological management or using another class of drug that poses less risk.
♦ Make sure patients at risk are made aware of warning signs and reviewed regularly.
♦ In very complex cases, talk to a colleague or pharmacist to help assess the risk/benefit ratio of prescribing and possible options.

Think about...

Developing your knowledge further by working through the Clinical Knowledge Summary (CKS) available on the NICE website on ADRs: https://cks.nice.org.uk/adverse-drug-reactions. This covers the practical aspects of assessing and managing a reaction as well as reporting the ADR.

Reporting ADRs

It is vital that all those working in healthcare engage with reporting of ADRs as part of what is called post-marketing surveillance. This means that all drugs are intensively monitored after they come on to the market and any suspected ADRs should be reported to the MHRA. These new drugs can be identified in the BNF as they have a black triangle next to the drug name. This black triangle usually stays in place for five years, but this can be extended if there are any concerns about the medication. The reason for this monitoring is that the clinical trials that drugs go through before being granted a product licence will only ever identify some of the ADRs that may happen when a patient takes a drug. There are occasions where medicines have been withdrawn from the market because ADRs not picked up in the clinical trials were reported in practice by clinicians.

Potential ADRs should be reported to the MHRA via the yellow card scheme. This can be done in a variety of ways, including online. It can also be done by the patient themselves. There are certain criteria about what and when to report. Find out how to do this so that when you have a patient present with an ADR, you know what to do.

Think about...

♦ Identifying particular drugs or patient groups that you will be encountering that are at high risk of developing ADRs.
♦ How you think you will identify and manage ADRs in your area of practice?
♦ Do you know what, when and how to report an ADR?
♦ Whether you know what a black triangle drug is and when you should report these (if you don't, then go to https://www.gov.uk/drug-safety-update/the-black-triangle-scheme-or to find out).

Individual Patient Variation: Pharmacogenetics

Not all patients are the same and you will be familiar with this in terms of things such as their medical history or pre-disposition to certain conditions. What you may not be aware of, however, is that the way patients handle drugs can vary depending on genetic factors. The branch of pharmacology that focuses on this is known as pharmacogenetics.

There is significant interest in how this can be used in the future to tailor medicines to patients depending on their genetic makeup. It may well be within your career that this is something that will become part of routine practice. For now, however, it is enough to be aware that genetic variation can affect certain drugs used in practice.

One way is through variable metabolism of drugs. Codeine is one important example. This drug is metabolised by CYP450 isoform CYP2D6. There is a significant inter-patient variation in the production of this isoform, meaning that the rate of codeine metabolism varies widely between patients. As codeine is a prodrug that is metabolised to the active metabolite morphine, this means that the therapeutic response also varies widely. Patients are categorised by their ability to metabolise codeine as either poor metabolisers or extensive metabolisers.

- **Poor metabolisers of codeine**: reduced therapeutic effect due to reduced ability to metabolise codeine into morphine.
- **Extensive metabolisers of codeine**: increased levels of morphine mean there is a risk of adverse effects, such as drowsiness and respiratory depression.

Conclusion

In this chapter we have covered a lot of different topics and hopefully you now have a greater understanding of the range of ways in which individual patients can respond to medicines differently. Your confidence and ability to tailor treatment will grow with your knowledge and experience. It is important to take the opportunity to focus on any groups that you will be working with during your independent prescribing training. The references and further reading included below will hopefully give you a starting point for building this knowledge and experience. One of the key factors in safe and effective prescribing is knowing where to find the information you need, as you will not remember everything straight away. Making sure you build up an awareness of where to find this information will support you in being as safe and effective as possible when you start out as a prescriber.

Key Points of This Chapter

- No patient is the same; the skill is to be able to assess the patient in front of you and apply your pharmacology knowledge to that person.
- If you know the basic principles of pharmacology, these will help you to identify those patients who may handle drugs differently.
- It takes time to build up knowledge and experience of working with specific patient groups, so make sure you invest this time in those areas within your scope of practice.
- It is also important to build up your knowledge of where to find the information and support you will need when you initially begin prescribing.

References and Further Reading

Aronson, J.K. (ed.) (2006). *Meyler's Side Effects of Drugs: The international encyclopedia of adverse drug reactions and interactions*. Oxford: Elsevier.

Ashley, C. and Dunleavy, A. (2014). *The Renal Drug Handbook: The ultimate prescribing guide for renal practitioners*, 4th ed. London: Radcliffe Publishing.

British National Formulary (BNF). *British Medical Association and Royal Pharmaceutical Society of Great Britain*. (Regular updates are published every quarter – make sure you use the most up-to-date edition or use the online version available on the NICE website.)

British National Formulary for Children (BNFC) (2018). *British Medical Association and Royal Pharmaceutical Society of Great Britain*. (As with the other version, regular updates are published every quarter – make sure you use the most up-to-date edition or use the online version available on the NICE website.)

Davey, P., Wilcox, M., Irving, W. and Thwaites, G. (2015). Prescribing in special groups: effects of age, pregnancy, body weight, and hepatic and renal impairment. In *Antimicrobial Chemotherapy*. Oxford: Oxford University Press.

Dodds, L.J. (2013). *Drugs in Use: Clinical case studies for pharmacists*. London: Pharmaceutical Press.

Katzung, B., Masters, S. and Trevor, A. (eds) (2012). *Basic and Clinical Pharmacology*. Maidenhead: McGraw-Hill.

Kearns, G.L., Abdel-Rahman, S.M., Alander, S.W., Blowey, D.L., Leeder, S. and Kauffman, R.E. (2003). Developmental pharmacology: drug disposition, action, and therapy in infants and children. *New England Journal of Medicine*, 349: 1157–67.

Loebstein, R. Lalkin, A. and Koren, G. (1997). Pharmacokinetic changes during pregnancy and their clinical relevance. *Clinical Pharmacokinetics*, 33(5): 328–43.

Mangoni, A.A. and Jackson, S.H.D. (2004). Age-related changes in pharmacokinetics and pharmacodynamics: basic principles and practical applications. *British Journal of Clinical Pharmacology*, 57(1): 6–14.

Pavek, P., Ceckova, M., Staud, F., (2009) *Variation of drug kinetics in pregnancy*. Current Drug Metabolism. 10, 520–529.

Pirmohamed, M., James, S., Meakin, S., Green, C., Scott, A.K., Walley, T.J., Farrar, K., Park, B.K. and Breckenridge, A.M. (2004). Adverse drug reactions as cause of admission to hospital: prospective analysis of 18,820 patients. *British Medical Journal*, 329: 15–19.

Preston, C. (ed.) (2016). *Stockley's Drug Interactions*. London: Pharmaceutical Press.

Prosad, S.P., Whibley, J. and Paul, S. (2011). Challenges in paediatric prescribing. *Nurse Prescribing*, 9(5): 220–26.

Rang, H.P., Ritter, J.M., Flower, R.J. and Henderson, G. (2015) *Rang & Dale's Pharmacology*. London: Elsevier.

Schaefer, C., Peters, P., Miller, R.K. (eds) (2014) *Drugs During Pregnancy and Lactation: Treatment Options and Risk Assessment*. Oxford: Academic Press.

Weersink, R.A. et al. (2016). Evaluating the safety and dosing of drugs in patients with liver cirrhosis by literature review and expert opinion. *BMJ Open*, 6: 1–7.

Walker R., Whittlesea C. (eds) (2012). *Clinical Pharmacy and Therapeutics*. Oxford: Elsevier/Churchill Livingstone. (This contains good chapters on pharmacogenetics, ADRs, drug interaction, drugs in pregnancy and lactation as well specific therapeutic areas.)

World Health Organization (1972). *WHO Technical Report No 498*. Available at: http://apps.who.int/iris/handle/10665/40968.

Useful Websites

Clinical Knowledge Summaries from NICE on different clinical topics that can link to the topics covered in this chapter. Available at: https://cks.nice.org.uk/#?char=A.

The Electronic Medicines Compendium (eMC) is a database of the SPCs for medicines that are licensed in the UK. Available at: https://www.medicines.org.uk/emc.

Medicines for Children is a great website featuring information and advice in giving medicines to children. It provides information that can be shared with parents. Available at: https://www.medicinesforchildren.org.uk.

The MHRA provides information on medicines safety and is particularly useful for reporting of side-effects/ADRs. Available at: https://www.gov.uk/government/organisations/medicines-and-healthcare-products-regulatory-agency.

The National Institute for Clinical Excellence (NICE) includes guidance on various topics, such as managing ADRs, prescribing in renal disease. It is important to be aware of what guidance they have that may influence your practice as they are a national NHS body producing evidence based guidance. Available at: https://www.nice.org.uk.

NHS Specialist Pharmacy Services (SPS) is a website that has useful information on prescribing for staff working in the NHS. There are various articles that review evidence and aim to help prescribing decisions, particularly where there is limited evidence. Available at: https://www.sps.nhs.uk.

Chapter 10
Continuing Professional Development and Reflective Practice

Amanda Blaber, Graham Harris and Vince Clarke

In This Chapter

♦ Introduction
♦ Defining 'professional practice'
♦ Sources of expectations of a professional
♦ What constitutes 'advanced practice' for the paramedic profession?
♦ What is the purpose of reflection on your prescribing practice?
♦ Why write up reflections on your prescribing practice?
♦ Commonly cited barriers to written reflection
♦ Ideas on how to make your reflections meaningful
♦ Reflective models
♦ Reflexivity versus reflection
♦ Clinical supervision or person-centred development?
♦ Continuing professional development
♦ Key points of this chapter
♦ References and further reading
♦ Useful websites

Introduction

This chapter sets the context of professionalism in relation to advanced practice and your role as an independent prescriber. The chapter will concentrate on ways to commence reflection and integrate this into your everyday practice. As people, we reflect for a large majority of our day, usually without consciously recognising that we are doing so. As professionals, we reflect at the time of care giving or 'in action' as Schön suggests (1983), whilst deciding on our interpersonal approach and communication, assessment, treatment and destination. Our reflections affect our decision-making process and patient outcome. Much of this occurs automatically without us pausing and saying to ourselves 'now let me reflect'. We certainly think about people we have cared for after the event – 'reflection on action', as Schön (1983) suggests.

Reflection will be explored as an individual process, moving on to more group-centred activities. A brief overview of some reflective models will also be provided.

Reflection on practice is a key aspect of advancing practice and is an essential part of your continuing professional development (CPD). The inextricable nature of these two subjects means it makes sense to include them in one chapter.

Defining 'Professional Practice'

'Professionalism' is a word commonly used in respect of all healthcare professions. The attributes of a profession and process of professionalisation has been the subject of much debate by sociologists and psychologists and have evolved over time. It is generally agreed that in order to be a 'legitimate' profession, there are several commonly agreed characteristics for any occupation to aspire to in order to use the term 'profession':

- To have their own specialised body of knowledge and related theories, gained through a higher education route.
- Having control, autonomy and accountability to define boundaries and the nature of work.
- Having a code of ethics which regulates relationships both between professions and professionals and their clients.
- Having a monopoly on their area of practice, i.e. no other health professional is able to perform the role.

The ongoing process of 'professionalisation' of the paramedic reflects the points made above. Professionalism is an interesting debate, which probably raises more questions than can be answered. For example:

Are roles within healthcare, like that that of an advanced paramedic, developing in complexity/diversity to satisfy societal demands of what the public expect healthcare professionals to be able to do?

Are advanced paramedics being utilised to 'plug the gap' for not enough doctors?

Are allied healthcare professionals who are not doctors being used as a source of cheaper labour?

Are advanced roles being developed to progress the professionalisation of the paramedic profession?

And so the questions go on, with interesting social and professional debates to be had. The debate is worth initiating to ensure the paramedic profession is clear about future progress and developments.

Certainly paramedics employed in advanced roles and those outside traditional ambulance employment are at the forefront of challenging role boundaries and are continuing to define 'professional practice'.

Sources of Expectation as a Professional

Using the term 'professional' comes with certain expectations of you as a registered healthcare professional (Jasper and Rosser, 2013). There are numerous sources that have specific expectations of you as a 'professional'; see **Box 10.1**.

Box 10.1 – Sources of professional expectation

1. The government –via social, health and economic policy which determines a paramedic's role.
2. The legal system – as the profession is regulated by law, paramedics are required to act lawfully, both personally and professionally.
3. Employers – who decide organisational roles.
4. Service users – who have expectations and first-hand experience of how paramedics act and execute their duties.
5. The general public and medics – who are responsible for constructing an image of the profession.
6. Colleagues – who set the culture by their own practice and actions, becoming role models for those entering the profession.
7. Other professions – who have their own views on the roles and functions of paramedics.
8. Registering bodies – the HCPC, who provide many publications that registrants are required to understand and abide by. An example of a few paramedic specific documents are:
   Standards of Proficiency: Paramedics (2014)
   Standards for Prescribing (2016b)
9. Professional body – College of Paramedics who work on behalf of their members to move the profession forward. (Website: www.collegeofparamedics.co.uk.)

As a registrant and advanced practitioner, you should know what the characteristics of a profession are and should meet the expectations that are incumbent upon you as a registered paramedic. This includes demonstrating the knowledge, skills and behaviours expected of you as a registered paramedic in a professional role. As an independent prescriber, you should ensure that you are fully cognisant of your professional practice responsibilities, which is why this chapter has briefly reviewed what 'professional practice' means. The parameters described in **Box 10.1** provide guidance for a practitioner's professional development. Points 1–9 in **Box 10.1** may act as a starting point for analysing practice, identifying good practice and assessing your own development needs.

Any professions standards and codes are broad in nature and attempt to be 'all encompassing' of all given situations that the professional may find themselves in. It can be argued that standards and codes may be quite restrictive for a professional working within an advanced scope of practice. The potential is for professional inertia. Staff working in the National Health Service (NHS) are familiar with the 6 Cs, with courage and compassion urged to be at the forefront of our practice and decision making, yet on occasions this is juxtaposed with restrictive professional standards. It is clear that the professional bodies are acting in the best interests of the public and professionals they represent. However, the more 'advanced' the professional becomes the more professional opinion, knowledge, experience, expertise and a whole host of other aspects are part of their everyday decision making. Professionalism is about working within your professional scope, whilst also being brave enough to select the best option for your patient and society.

A particularly pertinent aspect of advanced paramedic practice is the professional decision making **not** do something in any given situation. Advanced practitioners and independent prescribers use their knowledge, experience and expertise in all situations to make the best decision for their patient. In some cases, this will not involve skills application or prescribing. As some of the previous chapters have highlighted, knowing when not to prescribe is equally, if not more, important than the action of prescribing.

Before discussing several ways you may wish to consider in terms of how to do this, it is worth exploring the concept of 'advanced practice' from a paramedic perspective

 Turn to **Chapter 5** for further information on decision-making

What Constitutes 'Advanced Practice' for the Paramedic Profession?

On a national basis in the UK, advanced practice is acknowledged as that which requires the paramedic to have completed a relevant master's degree. Studying at Masters degree level (or level 7) challenges the individual to explore their practice area and associated subject complexities and is a fundamental requirement of a professional moving towards working clinically in an advanced practice role. Advanced clinical practice is characterised by a high degree of autonomy and complex decision making, and encompasses the four pillars of clinical practice, leadership and management, research and development, and education, along with the demonstration of core capabilities and area-specific clinical competence. It is clear that a paramedic applying for a prescribing course should possess a Masters degree qualification. Or as a minimum, be enrolled on a Masters degree pathway which includes a prescribing module within its structure.

The *Post-Registration – Paramedic career framework* (College of Paramedics, 2018) states that 'education for paramedic prescribing should be undertaken at level 7', and therefore where a full master's-level advanced practice award has not yet been achieved, prescribing would not normally be undertaken at the start of an advanced practice education pathway.

Together with this level of academic standing comes self-awareness, supporting colleagues and advancing the profession. There are more aspects to advanced practice, but in order to be an effective advanced practitioner, many people find the process of reflection essential. The next section will propose some potential useful 'self-help' ways to commence or continue your reflective abilities.

What is the Purpose of Reflection on Your Prescribing Practice?

Professional practice is full of dilemmas. The practitioner negotiates their way through these dilemmas on a daily basis, some are more simple than others, Schön (1987:1) describes the situation perfectly:

"In the varied topography of professional practice, there is a high, hard ground overlooking a swamp. On the high ground, manageable problems lend themselves to solutions through the use of research based theory and technique. In the swampy lowlands, problems are messy and confusing and incapable of technical solution. The irony of this situation is that the problems of the high ground tend to be relatively unimportant to individuals or society at large, however great their technical interest may be. While in the swamp lie the problems of greatest human concern. The practitioner is confronted with a choice. Shall he remain on the high ground where he can solve relatively unimportant problems according to his standards of rigor, or shall he descend to the swamp of important problems where he cannot be rigorous in any way he knows how to describe".

In some ways this refers back to the earlier discussion about expectations of a professional and professional body regulation. The question is what can professionals do about the 'swampy lowlands'? An aspiring advanced paramedic should be intrigued, engaged with and courageous enough to delve into the swampy lowlands. In these difficult situations, reflection is fundamental and an essential part of the process to 'tease' out the complexities, explore the possibilities, discover the truth about themselves, their colleagues and the profession to which they belong.

Think about...

How often would you say your 'thoughts or reflections' are meaningful?

Does just thinking about something help you personally?

Does reflecting upon something help you improve your care in the future?

Has reflecting on an incident or patient encounter ever helped you improve an outcome for a patient or helped you focus your own CPD?

Incidents/events 'bug' our heads, so writing may be a way for us to 'deal' with them effectively, professionally and developmentally. In any new role, professionals will naturally reflect more earlier on, until they feel they have worked through the 'novice' stage (Benner, 2000). Gradually becoming more confident and competent as learning progresses, the end point is that of 'expert' in this specific role. As a prescriber, you need to seriously consider using a structured written approach to reflection as one means of improving your practice. Perhaps the first step, if you are new to reflection, is to get started; some ideas follow in this chapter.

As healthcare professionals, it is usual that we are troubled by negative thoughts, but written reflection should also be used for positive outcomes and as a means to sharing best practice. As you will be aware, reflection is a means to assist the decision-making process, and can improve patient safety and quality of care. It forms a large part of paramedics' CPD requirements and can form a vital part of your own professional development if it is meaningful.

Why Write up Reflections on Prescribing?

As healthcare professionals, we recognise our responsibilities to record keep for ourselves and as part of our role in maintaining our patients' safety whilst in our care and beyond. However, we are often not good at writing about ourselves or our practice, which is equally important in our professional responsibility and development.

Writing a series of reflections as a newly qualified independent prescriber gives a permanence to your thoughts, feelings, practice and stage of development. This is more useful to you than transient thoughts, which are not recorded in any way. The passage of time means your thoughts are usually lost. What may eventually become a reflective experience may start as a series of practice or case notes, whilst you are working, an example of reflection-in action. It may be that you later wish, for your own personal development, to reflect more deeply on an aspect of your case notes, where a written reflection would be more suitable and become a more permanent and useful record.

Writing in a reflective way may end up becoming a mixture of formats, such as a reflective log (Jasper, 2008) or a structured account using a model. It depends on the purpose at hand as to which tool is most suitable. Your reflections may be nostalgic (for you to look back on years later), private or emotive, or may act as a form of communication to others, for example, via debrief. Written reflections can contribute to decision making if you encounter a similar situation again.

Commonly Cited Barriers to Written Reflection

There is a culture in many healthcare professions where anything to do with the practice should be undertaken in paid work time. It may be viewed that this culture is at odds with the concept of 'life-long learning' (HCPC 2014; 2016a). The process of life-long learning is not the employer's responsibility, but the registrants'. There will always be little or no time available in a working day for busy healthcare professionals to reflect effectively. The key word here is 'effectively'. We can think things through at the time or after the event, but are our efforts effective and reflective enough for us to truly say we have learnt from the experience or patient encounter? The ability of an individual to address their own shortcomings, lack of knowledge or learn from an experience depends on their own personal insight and self- awareness. We take advantage of learning opportunities as they come our way, across the course of a day, but there will be times when an individual wishes to spend more time after wards exploring, learning and reflecting on a specific aspect.

Many professionals cite 'time' as a barrier to reflecting. Some people may find it hard to accept that it may be worth spending some of their own time away from the working environment on meaningful reflection. To those people I would ask the following question: if something from your working day is 'bugging' your head, how much of your own time have you given it anyway? Would it have been a more efficient use of your 'downtime' to log, write a case study or write reflectively, which may have resolved your nagging doubts and questions? As already mentioned, means of reflection can take different forms and individuals need to explore what works best for them and suits the situation that requires exploring.

Ideas on How to Start Reflecting in a Meaningful Way

Many of us have been asked to write a written reflection as an academic piece of work at one time or another, which forms part of the assessment process. Some people will have found this process quite cathartic, while others may have found it annoying and not at all useful. Writing for an assessment is very different from writing for your own personal reasons, whether they be emotive or developmental.

You need to be ready to write reflectively; only you can see its benefits. Some key points that theorists on reflection, such as Rolfe et al. (2010), Bolton (2005; 2010), Jasper (2008 ; 2013) and Jasper et al. (2013) deem to be vital are as follows:

♦ Commitment from you is required in order to get the most from the reflective processit.
♦ You need to make time for yourself.
♦ It will work best if you are self-aware; this may require additional work (the NHS leadership academy website has some useful exercises).
♦ It cannot be undertaken quickly and results may not be immediate.
♦ You need to be 'honest and open' in your writing.
♦ You must want to learn from your experiences. Initially, when you begin to write you may find yourself out of your 'comfort zone'. You may also have this sense when you commence your role of independent prescriber. With more reflective writing, you may be able to recognise tangible results from yourself and professional exploration. This should enhance your prescribing practice.
♦ You may need to explore a subject in depth in order to achieve the level of understanding required of your new role as an independent prescriber and work towards becoming more confident and competent.

♦ During your depth of exploration, you may also explore your relationships inside and outside of the work environment, wider societal issues, and the culture of the health service and your profession. The reflective process should not be restrictive.

There will be times when you need to write reflections for academic or CPD purposes. It is not necessarily the purpose of this chapter to discuss reflection in relation to academic assessment. Many experts on reflective writing (Jasper et al., 2013; Bolton and Delderfield, 2018) agree that there are various strategies for reflective writing. They agree reflective writing can be described as a continuum, with analytical reflective writing at one end and creative writing at the other.

Analytical strategies are usually used when others are likely to see your writing. In such circumstances, 'models of reflection' may be used to come to an end action point. Other examples of analytical reflective writing strategies include:

♦ critical incident analysis
♦ using frameworks or models
♦ strengths, weaknesses, opportunities and threats (SWOT) analysis
♦ report writing
♦ learning outcomes
♦ journal writing/log.

Towards the more creative end of the reflective writing continuum are:

♦ writing to another
♦ writing unseen letters or emails
♦ storytelling/poetry.

The more creative the strategy used, the less analysis achieved generally. Creative examples may be useful if you are trying to initiate discussion with others on a subject or to capture your own unique version of an event. Which strategy you choose will depend on the following:

♦ Why you want to write – assessment or personal.
♦ Who is likely to see it – personal or public.
♦ What happened – personal or professional development.
♦ What do you want to achieve from the reflective experience?
♦ Is there anyone else involved?
♦ Are there any professional/ethical issues?

Below are some of the short-term goals that may help you get started on the reflective writing 'road' and for the outcome to be meaningful rather than functional.

Short-Term Reflection Ideas to Get You Started

If you perceive 'time' to be a barrier in reflecting, these ideas may help. Jasper and Mooney (2013) and Bolton (2018) believe that these techniques can be used on a daily basis and should not be seen as additional to your work. The point is to make a note of what happens during your day for potential reflective use at a later date. Below are two of their suggested techniques:

Three a day (Jasper and Mooney, 2013)

Think about and write down the three most important things that happened *to you* during a shift. If this becomes tedious, you can alter the focus, by considering what you enjoyed the most; what you enjoyed the least; what you learnt during the shift; what challenged you the most; things you did not know; things felt confident about; things you felt inadequate while doing; and things that did (or did not) go as planned. The list can keep growing – things that come into your head are the most important. Jotting them down during your shift may help when you reflect after it is over.

Time-limited stimuli (Bolton, 2018)

It may be hard at first. Set yourself a short period of time, say six minutes. Sit with a pen and paper, and write down whatever comes into your head. It appears that having to commit something to paper stimulates the brain to bring experiences to your mind from its depths. This can then form the basis of your reflection should you so wish.

Medium-Term Reflection Goals

Keep a reflective log or journal that you commit to writing once a week, making a pact with yourself to do so OR

Set time aside each week to review what has happened and record your feelings and reflections OR

Identify one event per week that stands out in your mind to explore in depth each week. You must be prepared to delve deeper into the experience and challenge yourself to learn more and view it from others' perspectives. Spend no longer than one hour per week on the above. If you are consistent and apply yourself, over time, all of these small 'chunks' will provide you with the following:

♦ Identification of your learning needs as an independent prescriber.
♦ Learning from your experiences.
♦ Developed action plans from your experiences.
♦ You may have solved problems in practice that have been around a while.
♦ A greater understanding of the way you work as a professional.
♦ You will have created an ongoing record of your development as an independent prescriber.

♦ You will have material that you can build on from a practice development perspective and may form the basis of problem-based learning with other colleagues who are experiencing the new role of prescribing for themselves.
♦ The creation of a professional portfolio in a gradual manner.
♦ You will have evidence of achieving your CPD standard.

Reflection is a process that is as important to a professional as other activities, such as record keeping or keeping up to date with developments in practice. It should be an integral part of who you are as an advanced paramedic and an independent prescriber.

Long-Term Reflection Goals

If you reach the stage of long-term goals, you will probably be in the 'habit' of reflecting and will find that it comes very naturally to you now and is part of who you are. One really simple way to continue your reflective writing is to review your previous writing. Over time and with your prescribing experience accumulating, reviewing your earlier reflections should be an interesting exercise, enabling you to clearly see your journey and your triumphs, and possibly allowing you to identify issues that were important back then and that may still be relevant. You may wish to use some of your writing to share with others or use it to stimulate discussion in a professional group situation. The writing that you wish to share will certainly form part of your professional portfolio.

Reflective Models

Remember, there are no rules in relation to reflection. It is yours. As mentioned earlier, reflective models are said to be useful when you require a structure and format for a reflective exercise, usually as part of an assessment process. A model approach may be useful for CPD or a portfolio presentation. The following sectionwill provide an overview of some commonly used models, with details of where to find more information on the specific model being given in the reference list at the end of the chapter (see **Table 10.1**).

Some of models in **Table 10.1** may be familiar. The table represents a small but varied selection of the numerous models that are available for you to use. The most important factor is that you take the time to research and find a model that suits you personally and suits the purpose for which you intend to use it.

Box 10.2 has used some of the sections/prompts that are advocated by the Council of Wales Deanery for GP prescribing CPD (2018) framework, and examples of the original framework can be found on their website (see the references section for details). However, the prescribing framework presented in **Box 10.2** has been developed to be more suited to the early career prescriber.

Box 10.2 provides a suggested means for paramedics to begin reviewing their prescribing practice. It is hoped that paramedics will reflect on the medications they have prescribed for their patients on a regular basis in order to develop their

Table 10.1 – Examples of some models of reflection

Name	Year	Title	Key concepts
Gibbs	1988	Reflective cycle	Six cyclical steps ♦ Description – what happened? ♦ Feelings – what were you thinking and feeling? ♦ Evaluation – what was good and bad about the experience? ♦ Analysis – what else can you make of the situation? ♦ Conclusion – what else could you have done? ♦ Action plan – if it arose again, what would you do?
Kolb	1984	Experiential learning theory	Works on two levels: four-stage cycle of learning and four separate learning styles Four-stage cycle of learning: ♦ Concrete experience or 'Do' – learner actively experiences an activity in practice ♦ Observation and reflection or 'Observe' – reflective observation – learner consciously reflects back on the experience ♦ Forming abstract concepts or 'Thinks' – learner attempts to conceptualise a theory or model of what is observed ♦ Active experimentation or 'Plan' – learner tries to plan how to test a model or theory or plan a forthcoming experience Four learning styles: ♦ Assimilators – learn better when presented with sound logical theories to consider ♦ Convergers – learn better when provided with practical application of concepts and theories ♦ Accommodators – learn better when provided with hands on experiences ♦ Divergers – learn better when allowed to observe and collect a wide range of information
Johns	1995	Model of reflection	Based on the work of Carper (1978) Five cue questions arranged cyclically: ♦ Description of the experience – describe it and identify the significant factors ♦ Reflection – what was I trying to achieve and what were the consequences? ♦ Influencing factors – what things like external/internal/knowledge affected my decision making? ♦ Could I have dealt with it better? What other choices did I have and what might have been their consequences? ♦ Learning – what will change because of this experience and how did I feel? How has this experience changed my ways of knowing: • empirics – scientific • ethics – moral knowledge • personal – self-awareness • aesthetics – the art of 'what we do', our own experiences Johns' textbook (2017) contains other useful healthcare-related ideas for reflective practice

Name	Year	Title	Key concepts
Bolton	2010	'Through the mirror' reflective practice writing model	Developed on the basis that all of our actions are founded upon our personal ethical values. 'We are what we do, rather than what we say we are.' (Bolton, 2010, p. 4)
			Writing 'through the mirror' is intuitive and spontaneous, like producing a first draft of an essay. These writings can then form the basis of discussion for confidential trusted forums or used by ourselves to learn more about who and what we are in practice. It provides insight into why we act as we do. The process can be unsettling and uneasy. It has been compared to mindfulness
			It is never good enough to say 'I don't have time to do X'; 'I did that because my senior told me to'. In healthcare and life in general, there is much that is out of our control. But we are all responsible for our own actions
			If the concepts of this model are embraced, it has the potential to help you explore and 'question everything, turning your world inside out, outside in and back to front' (Bolton, 2010, p. 11), hence the title 'through the mirror'
Ramsey	2005	Narrative learning cycle	Writing a story or narrative can provide some people who find reflection difficult with a way to express an experience with more confidence. Writing a story enables the use of 'she' or 'he' instead of 'I'. Some people will feel 'safer' and find this approach less personally revealing
			Fiction can slowly reveal episodes or combine things that happened at different times into one 'chunk' of writing. Your writing will still be from a deep professional experience and by 'retelling' may enable you to tackle issues 'head on', convey varying and various viewpoints (other than just your own), and may reduce anxiety about reflecting on a painful incident

prescribing practice and expertise. This framework provides prompts for the prescriber to consider during their reflection, which is important in roles that are new to an individual. As the prescriber becomes more competent, they will become less reliant on the prompts and will be able to reflect in their own unique way, probably using a recognised model of reflection.

Think about...

Are there any other prompts/questions that you would add to the framework in **Box 10.2?**

Box 10.2 – Paramedic prescribing reflective framework

Name of drug	
Mode of action	Route
Dose/duration	Specify dose and length of prescription
Pharmacology	How does this drug work?
	If a patient asks you 'how it works'/'what does it do', can you explain it?
	Review your associated anatomy and physiology
Why did I choose this drug?	Review your reasons
	Explore alternatives
What was I trying to achieve for this patient?	Review the patient's presenting complaint
	Review patient-specific issues, such as any other medication they may have been taking
	Consider possible drug interactions
Social history/considerations	Considerations which may have been affected or enhanced
	For example, prescribing diuretics to a person with limited mobility. It may be very difficult for them to get to the toilet as often as needed. Thus, this may result in them not being concordant with your prescription
Positives of your drug choice	
Negatives of your drug choice	
Learning points	Review what you have learnt from thinking about this patient encounter
Action plan	What do I need to know in order to prescribe more effectively next time?
	What do I need to learn?
	What can I read?
	Who can I talk to?

Reflexivity versus Reflection

In the course of your studies, you may hear the term 'reflexivity' mentioned. Experts on reflection provide clear definitions of the two, which are worth making clear in this chapter. Bolton (2010, p. 13) defines reflection as 'learning and developing through examining what we think happened on any occasion, and how we think others perceived the event and us, opening our practice to scrutiny by others, and studying data and texts from the wider sphere'.

Bolton (2010) suggests that reflexivity is somewhat deeper in terms of the reflective process and is more of an internal examination of us as individuals. This is perhaps one of the more meaningful definitions of reflexivity: 'What are the mental, emotional and value structures which allowed me to lose attention and make that error?' (Bolton, 2010, p. 14). This focus on the negative needs to be balanced with positive reflections and celebrations of good practice and positive experiences.

Bolton (2010) suggests that this deep questioning is omitted if the practitioner undertakes the reflective process as a problem-solving exercise of: what happened; why; what did I think and feel; and how can I do it better next time? Bolton suggests a 'through the mirror' model to assist practitioners with this self-exploration (see **Table 10.1**).

There are times in paramedic practice where discussing issues in a group situation is useful. The term 'debrief' is one that all emergency care workers are familiar with. However, the usefulness and success of such sessions vary enormously and may leave more unanswered questions and worries than they solve. Very often they are organised quickly, in response to an incident and run by an individual who does not have the facilitative expertise or experience. They may also be part of a 'tick box' exercise, on behalf of the organisation, to say that a debrief was conducted.

Think about...

How often are debriefs evaluated?

Do members of the group really have a chance, immediately after an incident, to reflect on what happened and explore their own feelings and role?

Other health professions have utilised the process of clinical supervision as a means to reflect, explore and be mindful about their practice in a small facilitated group environment. The next section of the chapter will explore clinical supervision and person-centred development (PCD) as an additional means of reflection, professional and personal development.

Clinical Supervision or Person-centred Development?

Historical Perspective and Moving from Clinical Supervision towards PCD

Clinical supervision was introduced into clinical practice in the 1920s. The aim was to facilitate PCD. Clinical supervision can occur on a one-to-one basis or as a small group, being supervised by one supervisor to facilitate proceedings. Hence, there is a relationship between the supervisor and the person(s) involved. This partnership should be of equal status between all parties and should not reflect any type of management hierarchy. The primary focus should be on the needs of the supervisee(s), but the needs of facilitator(s) should not be negated. In some situations, the supervisors also need support and require a means to have their needs 'facilitated'.

> **Definition**
>
> Elliott (2013, p. 174) defines clinical supervision as being 'about a supervisor facilitating supervisees to reflect on their past, present and future behaviour and its consequences'.

Purpose and Benefits

In many clinical areas, clinical supervision is embedded in practice. Many professionals find it an important part of their everyday work and rely on it in order to maintain their professional equilibrium, both physically and mentally. In other professions, the culture is not one of discussing, but of carrying on and 'doing'. Elliott (2013, p. 169) suggests that clinical supervision should be part of all healthcare organisation and should be happening as a matter of due course. It should be available to all, irrespective of their 'appointment, role or status'. The focus should definitely not be on corporate or management objectives.

However, the organisation will also benefit, as supervisees have more self-awareness and insight into their own practice. They may have more understanding of their accountability and potential to be fallible. For the organisation, this may translate into reducing adverse incidents involving patients and of staff taking greater professional accountability and responsibility for their own practice. More importantly, the patient should benefit from higher-quality care and a safer journey.

All writers on this subject (Elliott, 2013; Cassedy, 2010) warn of the danger of clinical supervision being facilitated by a line manager, where the process will then have managerial connotations. This is not how clinical supervision should be facilitated.

Key Features and Optimising Usefulness in Structure and Process

The following bullet points reflect the research of Winstanley and White (2003, p. 25), who found that clinical supervision is most effective, positive and productive if it includes:

- sessions around 60 minutes in length
- at least monthly sessions (if not more frequent)
- group sessions rather than one-to-one
- conducted away from the participants' workplace
- supervisor was selected by the participants rather than allocated to the role.

The role of supervisor should: encourage supervisees to challenge their own attitudes, values and beliefs; encourage supervisees to push the limits of their thinking; and question their own work-based activities and those of others in a professional manner. The clinical supervision process may have multiple benefits for individuals, which are summarised below:

- Reduction in stress levels, less risk of burnout and reduction in emotional stress.
- Improved self-awareness.
- Improved self-esteem.
- Improved confidence.
- Helping the person to reflect and think about their practice.
- Feeling more supported and valued.
- Improvement in the person's depth of knowledge and understanding.
- Enhanced personal and professional development.
- A greater sense of personal achievement and satisfaction at work.
- More confidence and support when challenging poor practice or behaviour of colleagues.

Care must be taken that the clinical supervision process does not become a means of staff 'surveillance' and is not seen in this way (Cassedy, 2010; Hawkins and Shohet, 2012). For paramedics, who very often do not find out the outcome of their patient's journey, clinical supervision may provide a means of support and practice discussion for what can be a lonely profession in some respects. However, as you can now appreciate, it is more than just a discussion about practice issues. The term 'clinical supervision' may provide a misleading understanding of the process, implying directing, controlling or watching over others. For many staff, clinical supervision has become imposed and prescriptive. Elliott (2013) argues that it is time to redefine the term and proposes the use of the term 'person-centred development'.

Person-Centred Development (PCD)

Advocates of PCD are clear that it has a universal meaning, which cannot be misunderstood or manipulated by employers:

Person – the individual
Centred – a focal point
Development – personal and professional growth, progress and advancement.

The process of 'PCD promotes personal and professional development. During the process it can also have a positive effect on the individual and can serve to facilitate physical, psychological and social wellbeing' (Elliott, 2013, p. 184). The words chosen imply a biopsychosocial approach, where physical, psychological and social aspects are of the utmost importance.

Role of the Facilitator

The PCD process should not include management in any form and it is inappropriate for facilitation to be conducted by a line manager or anyone holding a management position, especially if that manager is likely to be in a position where they may have a conflict of interest. Individuals should be able to choose their facilitator. If a new member of staff joins the organisation, the staff member should be supported if (at a later date) they decide they do not want the facilitator originally allocated to them.

The factors identified in **Table 10.2** will impact upon the PCD session. The outcome of a PCD session will therefore depend upon the facilitator's understanding and ability to integrate and apply the factors in order to achieve positive outcomes for the session. Some of the factors identified are things that we would assume are a 'given', but it is important for the facilitator to ensure that each of these are given equal importance and thought.

Role of the Participant

Individuals should be offered PCD, but should not be forced to take it. The facts of how the PCD approach is to be facilitated should be given so that individuals can make an informed decision and not be coerced. It is hoped that individuals will experience the benefit of PCD and value it as an option available to them. Also, the PCD process 'breeds' its own success, as participants find it valuable and a source of motivation to continue.

As a relatively new approach, PCD was initiated by Engle (1980) and developed by Ogden (2012), who identifies factors that can inform and impact on the PCD relationship of the facilitator and the participant, as identified in **Table 10.2**. It can be seen that many of the factors identified as important are directly relevant to healthcare workers and are specifically pertinent to paramedics.

Consideration is given to the majority of the factors in **Table 10.2**. The facilitator should be prepared to manage potentially difficult situations. For example, if a participant is fatigued, they are more likely to misinterpret or miscommunicate what is being said or the way they communicate, whether verbally or non-verbally. Thus, a facilitator needs to be prepared to resolve any such miscommunication. The ethos behind PCD is more holistic in nature and more of a partnership between the facilitator and the individual, and between the participants within the group.

The success of PCD can also be affected by the culture, age and gender of the individuals present at the PCD session. The attitude of participants will affect the success of the approach, as will their understanding of the purpose of the session. Participants must be assured that their workload will be covered during the PCD sessions. Participants who have a sense that they are needed 'back at work' will understandably, find it difficult to focus their attention during sessions.

Table 10.2 – Factors that can inform and impact on the PCD relationship

Physical aspects	Time of day
	Workload
	Identifying a dedicated time for PCD to occur and not be routinely cancelled
	Physical fatigue
	Hunger/thirst
	Comfort – seating, body space
	Environment – room allocated, temperature, lighting, ventilation
	Linking PCD sessions to duty rotas
	Flexible working
Psychological aspects	Degree of stress/anxiety
	Sense of personal safety
	Attitudes
	Freedom of choice
	Sense of acceptance into the group
	Sense of belonging
	Freedom from ridicule
	Feeling valued
	Past experience of group sessions
	Mood
	Motivation
	Communication – verbal, non-verbal
	Promotion of self-esteem
Social aspects	Confidentiality
	Establishing agreed-upon ground rules of the group
	Provision of education aimed at PCD and dissemination of information to all employees
	Sense of equality
	Facilitation, not dictation
	Self-expression
	Personal gain
	Maintaining dignity
	Receiving appropriate information

Think about...

As advanced practitioners and independent prescribers, maybe a fresh approach to providing yourselves with support in your new role is what is required.

Maybe PCD may provide you as a 'group of prescribers' with a way forward to personal and professional development.

It is perfectly possible for each of you to take on the role of facilitator on a rotational basis and discussing if this works for you all.

This chapter will now move on to discuss your CPD as an independent paramedic prescriber. See the 3rd edition of *Foundations for Paramedic Practice: a theoretical perspective* for details on your post registration CPD responsibilities and review Health and Care Professions Council (HCPC) (2017). *Continuing Professional Development and Your Registration.* London: HCPC.

Continuing Professional Development (CPD)

Undertaking CPD, sometimes termed Continuing Personal and Professional Development (CPPD), is an expectation of the majority of professional groups and a requirement laid down by most regulators of such groups. In the case of paramedics, the requirements for CPD are set by the HCPC and are presented as 'standards'. All HCPC registrants agree to undertake CPD as part of their ongoing registration and commit to such when completing their registration renewal declaration. A failure to maintain CPD standards may actually result in a fitness to practise concern being raised.

The formal HCPC CPD audit process began for paramedics in 2009, when the first tranche of paramedics' profiles were submitted and assessed. A random selection of 2.5% of registrants are selected for audit in each two-yearly cycle, meaning that the chances of being audited are low, but it is an expectation of the registered paramedic that they are meeting the standards regardless of whether or not they are audited.

If you are selected to submit your CPD profile, it will be reviewed by two assessors to see if you have met the five Standards. The audit cycle from 2013 to 2015 saw 430 paramedics selected for audit, with 79 being required to submit further information. This represents approximately 18% of selected profiles not meeting the Standards at the first submission for this period. In the audit cycle from September 2015 to September 2017, 597 paramedics were selected by the HCPC for audit. Eighty-seven of the selected paramedics, approximately 15%, did not meet the Standards at the first attempt and were required to submit further information. The remaining 85% of paramedics presented CPD profiles which met the Standards at the first submission (HCPC, 2016a).

Therefore, the trend is one which indicates that paramedics are becoming more proficient at demonstrating how they meet the HCPC's Standards for CPD.

There is a great deal of information regarding CPD on the HCPC website, which will not be repeated here. The aim of this section is to contextualise the HCPC CPD expectations in the context of the prescribing paramedic. To do so first requires a clarification of the HCPC Standards, as detailed in **Box 10.3**.

Box 10.3 – HCPC Standards for CPD

A registrant must:

1. Maintain a continuous, up-to-date and accurate record of their CPD activities
2. Demonstrate that their CPD activities are a mixture of learning activities relevant to current or future practise
3. Seek to ensure that their CPD has contributed to the quality of their practice and service delivery
4. Seek to ensure that their CPD benefits the service user
5. Upon request, present a written profile (which must be their own work and supported by evidence) explaining how they have met the Standards for CPD.

Source: Health and Care Professions Council (2017). *Continuing Professional Development and Your Registration*. London. HCPC.

The main point to consider when approaching your CPD is that it must be relevant to *your* role. There are not separate or different expectations of the prescribing paramedic in the same way as there are not differing standards for paramedics working in primary care or those in education. As a paramedic, your CPD profile will be expected to meet the generic HCPC standards with the choice of activities reflecting your work setting and scope of practice.

In order to meet the Standards, you should make certain that you are accurately recording all of your CPD activities. If you have not yet done so, start now! You may choose to use a notebook, a computer spreadsheet or an online platform to do this, but remember that you are individually responsible for keeping these records safe and up to date. Your employer, whilst having a duty to maintain your statutory updates, is NOT responsible for your CPD. As a registered healthcare professional, it is your responsibility to keep up to date and seek out appropriate methods of doing so. If you have the support (either financial or time-related) of your employer, then that is a bonus.

The HCPC accepts both digital and hard-copy profiles, so keeping an electronic copy may make submission to the HCPC's online submission portal easier in the future.

Box 10.4 sets out some guidance on how and what to record as you undertake your CPD activities with a specific view to meeting the expectations of the HCPC CPD assessors.

Box 10.4 – Meeting Standard 1

♦ Make a list of your CPD activities as you complete them.
♦ Record all of your CPD activities regularly and frequently. Set aside some time to work on your CPD record every few weeks.
♦ Be accurate in your recording. Note the actual date that you undertook an activity rather than the month or period. This demonstrates that you have been completing your list as you have done your CPD rather than retrospectively at the end of a two-year period!
♦ Note as much information as possible about the activities that you complete. Using the headings below will help you to record all of the most useful information as you go:
   • Date
   • Times
   • Activity
   • Type of Activity
   • Standard 3
   • Standard 4
♦ Record the date of each activity in chronological order. This allows the assessors to easily check your activity list for any significant gaps – you MUST NOT have any unexplained gaps of greater than three months.
♦ Record the details and the type of CPD activity. This allows the assessors to easily identify the type of activities that you are undertaking as well as seeing that you are undertaking a mixture of activities.
♦ Make brief notes about your CPD activities with Standards 3 and 4 in mind. This will demonstrate to the assessors that you have carefully considered the impact of your CPD.

A review of the HCPC guidance will show you that 'CPD is not only formal courses but any activity from which you learn and develop'. Unlike many regulatory or professional bodies, the HCPC does not set a 'points' or 'hours'-based CPD requirement; instead, it leaves it up to the individual to carry out CPD that they consider appropriate for themselves, focusing on an outcomes-based approach.

Such an approach can be a double-edged sword: on the one hand, it can be seen to give registrants the freedom to choose the type and amount of CPD that they undertake; on the other hand, it can be seen as lacking in sufficient direction and measurable, quantifiable outcomes for registrants to meet, with any activity having the potential to be presented as CPD.

The main point to remember is the outcome, i.e. does your CPD activity, whatever it might be, contribute to the quality of your practice and service delivery (Standard 3) and benefit the service user (Standard 4)?

To help you better understand the breadth of approaches, the HCPC sets out five categories of CPD: work-based learning, professional activity, formal education, self-directed learning and 'other'. Standard 2 states that registrants should: 'demonstrate that their CPD activities are a mixture of learning activities relevant to current or future practice.' In this context, 'mixture' simply means 'more than one'.

In the context of the prescribing paramedic, you may choose to reflect on a particularly challenging case or undertake a course which develops your understanding of a specific aspect of pharmacology.

Box 10.5 – Examples of CPD activities for prescribing paramedics

Work-based learning:

Reflecting on experiences at work: you might do this by making some informal notes or by writing up a more structured reflection following a recognised cycle or model. Either approach is acceptable as evidence of CPD.

Professional activity:

Being part of a prescribing steering group or similar that considers the wider impact of your role. Copies of meeting notes or minutes could be used as evidence.

Formal education:

Doing a course: if you use course attendance as an example of CPD, remember to identify how this has met Standards 3 and 4. Collecting certificates of attendance only goes part of the way to meeting the standards of CPD. Remember that your activities need to be a mixture. If you are undertaking a long-term course, such as a higher degree, you should avoid presenting this as your only activity. Instead, think of the different activities which you have undertaken within the course.

Self-directed learning:

Reading articles or books: keep a log of the books or articles that you have read and identify what influence they have had on your practice in relation to Standards 3 and 4. Your notes do not need to be extensive or follow a formal format, nor do you need to make notes on everything that you read.

Other:

Relevant public service or voluntary work: assisting with scouting, church, school, charity or sporting activities can be considered as CPD. Think about what qualities and abilities are being developed by your doing these activities and how they can be used in your professional role to meet Standards 3 and 4. As before, record how these Standards are being met by undertaking this activity using a template.

A key point to remember is that neither the HCPC nor your employer is able to demand that you share your entire CPD portfolio with them. The HCPC asks only for evidence of CPD by way of a written profile submission, which includes details of activities, personal statements and evidence. You are only required to submit examples of your CPD, not your entire CPD portfolio. The same situation should be true for employers.

This should give you some reassurance if you are compiling personal reflective accounts in which you identify how you felt about incidents and how you may adapt your practice in the future. You must, however, ensure that any information that you do keep as evidence meets any relevant data protection requirements and is fully anonymised.

For prescribing paramedics, your employer may not be used to employing paramedics or familiar with the professional regulation undertaken by the HCPC. Therefore, they may have requirements for an hours-based CPD element to be completed as part of your employment. In these circumstances, it is suggested that you maintain a single portfolio to meet the requirements of both the HCPC and the employer.

Conclusion

The concept of reflection has been explored. This chapter has provided some useful and varied ideas to help the clinician develop their ability to reflect in a more meaningful way. Reflection is very much a personal aspect of professional practice, where 'one size will not fit all' and therefore, this chapter has presented a mixture of approaches. Person-centred development has been explored, with some ideas on how this may be applied to paramedic prescribing practice. Finally, this chapter has explored the notion of professional practice in relation to CPD and the role/requirements of the HCPC.

Key Points of This Chapter

- Understanding the connotations and expectations of professional practice should contribute to your advanced prescribing practice.
- Reflection is an important part of both personal and professional development.
- Self-awareness, willingness to be honest and open, and persistence are the key to reflecting effectively.
- Various reflective models exist. These may be useful to provide structure and direction to the reflective process.
- Person-centred development is a more recent approach, designed to explore biopsychosocial aspects of a professionals role and may be more beneficial than clinical supervision.
- CPD is part of your role and responsibilities as a health professional.

References and Further Reading

Benner, P. (2000). *From Novice to Expert: Excellence and power in clinical nursing practice*. Upper Saddle River, NJ: Prentice Hall.

Blaber, A.Y. (2018). *Blaber's Foundations of Paramedic Practice: A theoretical perspective*, 3rd ed. London: Open University Press/McGraw-Hill.

Bolton, G. (2005). *Reflective Practice: Writing and professional development*, 2nd ed. London: Sage.

Bolton, G. (2010). *Reflective Practice: Writing and professional development*, 3rd ed. London: Sage.

Bolton, G and Delderfield, R. (2018). *Reflective Practice: Writing and professional development*, 4th ed. London: Sage.

Bulman, C. and Schutz, S. (eds) (2013). *Reflective Practice in Nursing*, 5th ed. Chichester: John Wiley & Sons.

Carper, B. (1978). Fundamental patterns of knowing in nursing. *Advances in Nursing Science*, 1(1): 13–23.

Cassedy, P. (2010). *First Steps in Clinical Supervision: A guide for healthcare professionals*. Maidenhead: Open University Press/McGraw-Hill.

College of Paramedics (2018). *Post-Registration – Paramedic career framework*. Bridgwater: College of Paramedics.

Council of Wales Deanery (2018). CPD for General Practitioners. Available at: https://gpcpd.walesdeanery.org/index.php/reflecting-on-prescribing.

Downie, J. (1989). *Professional Judgement: The getting of judgement*. Milton Keynes: Open University Press.

Elliott, P. (2013). Moving from clinical supervision to person-centred development: a paradigm change. In M. Jasper, G. Mooney and M. Rosser (eds), *Professional Development, Reflection and Decision Making in Nursing and Healthcare*, 2nd ed. Chichester: Wiley Blackwell.

Engle, G.L. (1980). The clinical application of the biopsychosocial model. *American Journal of Psychiatry*, 137: 525–44.

Gibbs, G. (1988). *Learning by Doing: A guide to teaching and learning methods*. Oxford: Further Education Unit, Oxford Polytechnic.

Hawkins, P. and Shohet, R. (2012). *Supervision in the Helping Professions*, 4th ed. Maidenhead: Open University Press/McGraw-Hill.

Health and Care Professions Council (HCPC) (2014). *Standards of Proficiency – Paramedics*. London: HCPC.

Health and Care Professions Council (HCPC) (2016a). *2013–15 Continuing Professional Development Audit Report*. London: HCPC.

Health and Care Professions Council (HCPC) (2016b). *Standards for Prescribing*. London: HCPC. Available at: http://www.hcpc-uk.co.uk/assets/documents/10004160Standardsforprescribing.pdf.

Health and Care Professions Council (HCPC) (2017). *Continuing Professional Development and Your Registration*. London: HCPC.

Jasper, M. (2008). Learning journals and diary keeping. In C. Bulman and S. Schutz (eds), *Reflective Practice in Nursing*, 4th ed. Chichester: John Wiley & Sons.

Jasper, M. (2013). *Beginning Reflective Practice*, 2nd ed. Cheltenham: Nelson Thornes.

Jasper, M. and Rosser, M. (2013). Practising as a professional. In M. Jasper, G. Mooney and M. Rosser (eds), *Professional Development, Reflection and Decision Making in Nursing and Healthcare*, 2nd ed. Chichester: Wiley Blackwell.

Jasper, M. and Mooney, G.,. (2013). Reflective writing for professional development. . In M. Jasper, G. Mooney and M. Rosser (eds), *Professional Development, Reflection and Decision Making in Nursing and Healthcare*, 2nd ed. Chichester: Wiley Blackwell.

Jasper, M., Mooney, G. and Rosser, M. (eds) (2013). *Professional Development, Reflection and Decision Making in Nursing and Healthcare*, 2nd ed. Chichester: Wiley Blackwell.

Johns, C. (1995). Framing learning through reflection within Carper's fundamental ways of knowing in nursing. *Journal of Advanced Nursing*, 22: 226–34.

Johns, C. (2017). *Becoming a Reflective Practitioner*, 5th ed. Oxford: Wiley Blackwell.

Kolb, D.A. (1984). *Experiential Learning: Experience as the source of learning and development*. Upper Saddle River, NJ: Prentice Hall.

Ogden, J. (2012). *Health Psychology: A textbook*, 5th ed. Maidenhead: Open University Press/McGraw-Hill.

Ramsey, C. (2005). Narrating development: professional practice emerging within stories. *Action Research*, 3(3): 279–95.

Rolfe, G., Freshwater, D. and Jasper, M. (2001). *Critical Reflection for Nursing and the Helping Professions: A User's Guide*, 2nd ed. Basingstoke: Palgrave Macmillan.

Schön, D.A. (1983). *The Reflective Practitioner*. London: Temple Smith.

Schön, D.A., (1987) *Educating the Refelctive Practitioner*. San Franciso: Jossey-Bass.

Winstanley, J. and White, E. (2003). Clinical supervision models, measures and best practice. *Nurse Researcher*, 10(4): 7–38.

Useful Websites

College of Paramedics: www.collegeofparamedics.co.uk.

Health and Care Professions Council (HCPC): www.hcpc-uk.co.uk.

NHS Leadership Academy: www.leadershipacademy.nhs.uk.

Index